Nutrition as a Key to Covid-19 Resilience in India

Nutrition as a Key to Covid-19 Resilience in India

Editors

Dr Garima Upadhyay

Dr Richa Agrawal

GYAN

Published, 2021

Published by

Gyan Publishing House
5, Ansari Road
Daryaganj, New Delhi-110002
Phone: 011-47034999, 9811692060
www.gyanbooks.com
E-mail: books@gyanbooks.com

Printed at: Gyan Press, Delhi.

Cataloging in Publication Data—DK
Courtesy: D.K. Agencies (P) Ltd. <docinfo@dkagencies.com>

Nutrition as a key to Covid-19 resilience in India / editors, Dr Garima Upadhyay, Dr Richa Agrawal.
pages cm
Contributed articles.
ISBN 9788121220484 (HB)

1. Immunity—Nutritional aspects. 2. Immunity—Nutritional aspects—India. 3. COVID-19 (Disease)—Nutritional aspects. 4. COVID-19 (Disease)—Nutritional aspects—India. 5. Medicine, Ayurvedic. I. Upadhyay, Garima, editor. II. Agrawal, Richa (Nutrition & lifestyle coach), editor.

LCC QR182.2.N86N88 2021 | DDC 616.079 23

Contents

Preface

During this pandemic, we had an opportunity to interact with people from different backgrounds, specially working in the field of Food and Nutrition. There was a felt need to have a literature on impact assessment on our food and eating habits, which were drastically affected because of COVID-19. Keeping this in view, we thought it would have been better to collate the efforts of experts in the field of Food and Nutrition, so that different ideas can be collected and published in a form of book, which might contribute in enriching the academicians as well as practitioners in this field.

We were able to get good response and support from seasoned and young scholars who have contributed their thoughts and experience in this volume. We hope this effort might result in bridging the gap between theory and practice regarding the impact of COVID-19 on Food and Nutrition.

The present work has tried to take into account different dimensions of the fall out of COVID-19 on the dietary lifestyle of Indian society. To begin with:

Chapter 1 deals how to increase our immunity and reduce the oxidative stress caused by the virus. Role of antioxidants in reducing the negative effect of oxidation and enhancing the capability of our immune system. Antioxidants are present in various food ingredients and each food ingredient's antioxidant capacity is measured by its ORAC value and foods with high ORAC value are also focused.

Chapter 2 deals with the challenges to infant and young child feeding practices created during this pandemic and evidences/ recommendations which can be converted into general practices nationwide, for positive outcomes.

Chapter 3 emphasises on Ayurvedic *Ahara* with special reference to pre-conception and pregnancy and its holistic management. Ayurveda gives prime importance to the preventive aspect and elaborates pre-conception and pregnancy diet for best quality progeny then and now even during pandemic.

Chapter 4 discusses on Food Security Status of India, Impact of COVID-19 on Food Security and Management Strategies from COVID-19 perspective.

Chapter 5 helps us to understand the role of Ayurvedic management in pandemic like Covid-19, it is essential to understand the concept of newly emerging disease, origin of epidemic/pandemic and mode of transmission of communicable diseases. The vitiated *dosha* (body humour) causes various disorders according to variation in *vikara-prakriti* (the natural course of disease), *samutthana* (etiological component) and *adhishthana* (location/ the site of pathological involvement). In *Sushruta Samhita*, the modes of human-to-human transmission of communicable diseases are mentioned as physical contact, exhalation, eating together in same plate, sharing bed, using clothes, garlands, and paste. Improper *ahara* (diet) and wrong *vihara* (behaviour) negatively influence healthy status of the body, mind, and sense organs. These concepts are very much relevant with the origin, disease spread, mode of transmission, disease severity and post-Covid impact. These all give a strong fundamental approach to understand epidemic/pandemic in Ayurveda and design management protocol accordingly.

Chapter 6 is based on the observation that several phytonutrients present in our daily diet can have the potential to fight against the disease. Many foods when tested against COVID-19 showed promising results. Phytonutrients such as polyphenols, vitamins and minerals like selenium and zinc have shown to provide protection from the virus by either acting as antiviral agents or as immunomodulators. In this chapter, role of some important functional foods and phytonutrients have been discussed which help in combating the disease.

Chapter 7 focuses on how synbiotic foods are boon to human health. Synbiotic is the right choice to meet the need of an hour, as they play an essential role in reducing the symptoms of the COVID-19 *i.e.,* respiratory and digestive problems. Synergistic products are the combination of pro and prebiotics, which helps in maintaining the gut health of the organism by enhancing the survival and implantation of live microbial food additives in the gastrointestinal tract, thereby stimulating growth and causing the metabolism of health- promoting bacteria, thus improving the health of host.

Chapter 8 This chapter summarises recent scientific literature on an optimal diet, vitamin and mineral supplementation, and good hygiene practices for food preparation during the COVID-19 pandemic. The findings can be used to help dietitians and healthcare professionals better address dietary recommendations during the COVID-19 pandemic. Guidance related to the safe handling of food, from production to consumption, is critical to reduce the risk of viral dissemination. The general recommendation is to consume a diet based predominantly on fresh foods such as fruits, vegetables, whole grains, low-fat dairy sources, and healthy fats (olive oil and fish oil) and to limit intakes of sugary drinks and processed foods high in calories and salt. Dietary supplements (i.e., vitamins C and D, zinc, and selenium) should be administered to individuals with, or at risk of, respiratory viral infections or in whom deficiency is detected. Breast milk is the safest and healthiest food for infants, and breastfeeding should be encouraged, even in women diagnosed with COVID-19.

Chapter 9 addresses critical health challenges, need of training of children to build immune systems, develop ability to fight off germs. Role of school environment and health education is also highlighted.

Chapter 10 provides a broad spectrum of information on the use of phytochemicals found in medicinal plants for the inhibition of corona virus family. Plant based foods are rich in Prebiotic which helps to improve our gut health and boost up immunity. Neutraceuticals acts as super food and provides better health with the combination of food and natural medicine. This chapter also provides a glimpse of little herbal food and its role in health. Green tea, flavonoids and polyphenols are very effective phytochemical which inhibits the growth of virus. Indian herbs and traditional foods are very rich in its medicinal importance. MERS, SARS, and COVID-19 are infectious disease and spread due to the virus. Plant based phytochemicals are helpful against virus thus protect us from infection. Many types of herbal medicines are beneficial for boosting immunity and fighting against the virus.

Dr Garima Upadhyay
Dr Richa Agrawal

List of Contributors

Dr Richa Agrawal, Ph.D (Food & Nutrition), BHU, Varanasi, Nutrition & Lifestyle Coach, Young & Fit, New Delhi

Dr Rachana Srivastava, Women Scientist, Department of Community Medicine and School of Public Health, Post Graduate Institute of Medical Education and Research, Chandigarh

Dr Poonam Khanna, Associate Professor, Department of Community Medicine and School of Public Health, Post Graduate Institute of Medical Education and Research, Chandigarh

Mr Savitesh Kushwaha, PhD Research Scholar, Department of Community Medicine and School of Public Health, PGIMER, Chandigarh-160012

Dr Anuradha Roy, Associate Professor,Department of Prasuti Tantra Faculty of Ayurveda, Institute of Medical Sciences, Banaras Hindu University, Varanasi

Dr Binay Sen, Assistant Professor Department of Dravyaguna, Faculty of Ayurveda, Institute of Medical Sciences, Banaras Hindu University, Varanasi

Dr Shachi Singh, Assistant Professor, Department of Botany, Mahila Mahavidyalaya, Banaras Hindu University, Varanasi

Dr Reena Verma, Assistant Professor, Department of Home Science, IIS (deemed to be University), Jaipur, Rajasthan

Dr Gargi Saxena, Senior Assistant Professor, Department of Home Science, IIS (deemed to be University), Jaipur, Rajasthan

Dr Priyanka, Assistant Professor, Department of Home Science, Vasant Kanya Mahavidyalaya Kamachha, Varanasi

Dr Sukanya Chakravorty, Assistant Professor, Department of Home Science, Mahila Mahavidyalaya, BHU, Varanasi

Dr Sangeeta, Assistant Professor, Home Science (Food & Nutrition), Ramabai Govt. Women P.G. College, Akbarpur- Ambedkarnagar.

1

Building Immunity through High ORAC Foods

Dr Richa Agrawal

Every struggling time provides the opportunity to learn something new.

Today the world is facing with Novel Corona virus which has severely affected the life of people. The deadly Virus has changed the way we work, interact or eat and thus the way we live. This virus especially infects the lungs resulting in oxidative stress which is fatal to our body.

Fight against the virus has made us understand the importance of boosting our immunity. We can take the preventive measure by increasing our immunity and reducing the oxidative stress caused by the Virus.

The ability of our body to defend against disease causing micro-organism is known as **Immunity**.

While our immune system is fighting against virus and bacteria, **Oxidation** takes place and creates inflammation resulting into cold, flu or weakness. In the process of oxidation, the oxygen molecules split up into single atom with unpaired electron. Electrons like to be in pairs, so these single atoms are called free radicals and they roam here and there to take electrons from other molecules in the body.

Free radicals, which are the end product of oxidation, are not absorbed by the body and they become harmful. Free Radicals are highly reactive compounds that attach and bind themselves to normal cells causing damage to cells, membranes and DNA while also leading to decreased immune response. Once free radicals are formed, a chain reaction occurs eventually affecting and damaging the whole cell. This cell damage can lead to various chronic degenerative diseases and pose severe health risks. For instance, Covid-19 affects respiratory system and induces oxidative stress in the body.

A strong immune system is the best weapon against such diseases and viruses.

Antioxidants play an important role in boosting immunity. Antioxidants are compounds that donate electrons to free radical within the body thus neutralising the negative effect of Free Radical Oxidation. Antioxidants are able to give an electron to a free radical without becoming destabilised themselves thus stopping the oxidation process and free radical chain reaction.

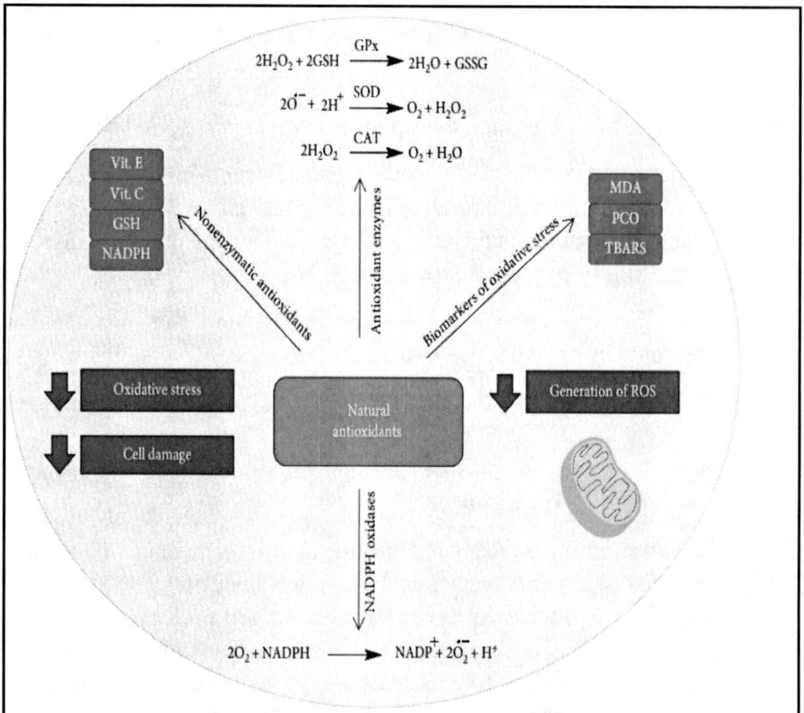

The main antioxidant mechanisms of natural compounds reported in this review. Dashed line: inhibition. Full line: activation.

Source: Hindawi, Oxidative Medicine and Cellular Longevity, Volume 2020, Article ID 3173281

Having understood the role of Antioxidants in reducing the negative effect of oxidation and enhancing the capability of our immune system it becomes important to increase the Antioxidant level in our body. Antioxidants are present in various food ingredients and each food ingredient's antioxidant capacity is measured by its ORAC value.

ORAC stands for 'Oxygen Radical Absorbance Capacity'. The ORAC unit is a method developed by scientists at the National Institute of Health and Aging (NIH) to measure the antioxidant capacity of different foods. It's a lab test that attempts to quantify the 'total antioxidant capacity (TAC)' of a food by placing a sample of the food in a test tube, along with certain other molecules that are vulnerable to oxidation. After a while they measure how well the sample protected the vulnerable molecules from oxidation by the free radicals.

The lesser is the damage by free radicals, the higher is the antioxidant capacity of the test substance. It is understood that foods with higher ORAC scores have greater antioxidant capacity.

ORAC value is an internationally recognised certified patented standard system and it is constantly developed based on research. It indicates the degree of Antioxidant capacity of the food.

Ingestion of 5000 (Five Thousands) ORAC units daily have been recommended by the United States Department of Agriculture (USDA).

Various studies have demonstrated that Herbs, Spices and Condiments possess the highest ORAC value compared to any other food ingredients.

Some of the Herbs, Spices and Condiments with the high ORAC values (in μmol TE/100g)

	ORAC VALUES	
Herbs, Spices & Condiments	***Unit in μmol TE/100g***	***Unit in μmol TE/10g***
Cinnamon (ground)	1,43,264	14,326
Cloves (Ground)	1,11,490	11,149
Turmeric (Ground)	44,776	4477
Peppermint (Fresh)	13,970	1397
Basil (Dried)	56,685	5668
Chilli Powder	21,827	2182
Cumin Seed	47,600	4760
Curry Powder	24,981	2498
Mustard Seed	28,759	2875
Black Pepper	10,205	1020
Coriander Leaves	5,141	514

Source: USDA Agriculture Research Service.

Extracts of Ginger, Tulsi (Basil) and Turmeric are atleast 10 times higher ORAC value and hence more effective. The higher ORAC values in the above Herbs, Spices and Condiments can majorly be attributed to available rich **Phytonutrients** in them. In the study Herbs and Spices have been identified as sources of various phytochemicals, many of which possess powerful antioxidant activity. These Phytonutrients have superior antioxidant properties. According to study it was observed that antioxidants in spices are a large group of bioactive compounds which consists of Flavonoids, Phenolic compounds, Sulphur-containing compounds, Tannins, Alkaloids, Phenolic diterpenes and Vitamins.

Phytonutrients are natural chemicals or bioactive compounds produced by plants. They have antioxidant and anti-inflammatory properties that can help support a strong immune system.

There are thousands of Phytonutrients found in plants and related foods. Some of the most important and common Phytonutrients are given in below Table.

Phytonutrients	*Type*	*Functions*	*Found in*
Carotenoids (Bright Coloured Hue)	Common Types		
	α carotene	Beneficial for Eye health & Immune health	Pumpkins, Carrots, Spinach, Kale, Oranges, Tomatoes
	β carotene		
	Crypto xanthin		
	Lutein		
	Lycopene		
	Zeo xanthin		
Ellagic Acid		Reducing cancer risk and lowering cholesterol	Strawberries, Raspberries, Grapes, Pomegranates, Walnuts
Resveratrol		This compound supports cardio-vascular & cognitive health. It increases cerebral blood flow	Predominantly in Grapes, specifically in Grape wine, Peanuts, Pistachio, Blueberry, Dark chocolate, Strawberries
Flabinoids	Flavones	This compound is rich in antioxidant molecules & anti - cancer properties	Green Tea, Apples, Onions, Coffee, Legumes, Ginger
	Anthocyanines		
	Flavanones		
	Isoflavones		
	Flavonols		
Phytoestrogens		Reducing the risk of cancer, heart disease and osteoporosis. Helps women in relieving discomfort from hot flushes and other menopausal symptoms	Soyabean, Broccoli, Oranges, Carrots, Coffee, Legumes.
Glucosinolates		Regulates inflammation, metabolic function and stress responses. Helps in cancer prevention	Cruciferous vegetables, Broccoli, Cauliflower, Mustard seed and Brussel spout

Below table summarises the available phytonutrients in various Spices and Herbs

Chemical composition of spices (seasonings) and culinary herbs [1, 3, 8]

Spices and Herbs	*Important Chemical Constituents*
Cloves	Eugenol, isoeugenol, acetyleugenol, sesquiterpene, pinene, vanillin, gallic acid, flavonoids, phenolic acids
Cinnamon	Eugenol, limonene, terpineol, catechins, proanthocyanidins, tannins, linalool, safrole, pinene, methyleugenol, benzaldehyde
Cardamon	Limonene, 1,8-cineole, terpinolene, myrcene, caffeic acid, quercetin, kaempferol, luteolin, pelargonidin
Coriander	Linalool, borneol, geraniol, terpineol, cumene, pinene, terpinene, quercetin, kaempferol, caffeic, ferulic, n-coumaric and vanillic acids, rutin, tocopherols, pyrogallol
Saffron	Crocins (water soluble carotenoids), safranal, flavonoids, gallic, caffeic, ferulic, *n*-catechuic, syringic, salicylic, and vanillic acids
Turmeric	Curcumins, essential oils, eugenol, carotene, ascorbic acid, caffeic, *p*-coumaric, protocatechuic, syringic, vanillic acid
Ginger	Gingerol, turmeric, paradol, geraniol, geranial, borneol, linalool, camphene, zingerol, zingiberon
Anise	Camphene, pinene, linalool, *trans*-, *cis*-anetholes, eugenol, acetanisole, rutin, luteolin-7-glucoside, apigenin-7-glucoside, isoorientin
Caraway	Monoterpenes, sesquiterpene, aromatic aldehydes, terpene esters, terpenol, terpenal, terpenon, limonene, safranal, kaempferol, quercetin, tannins, caffeic, ferulic, *p*-coumaric, and chlorogenic acids
Fenugreek	Sesquiterpenes, aromatic aldehydes, terpenes
Black pepper	Piperine, pinene, camphene, limonene, terpenes, piperidine, isoquercetin, sarmentine
Oregano	Apigenin, quercetin, luteolin, myricetin, diosmetin, eriodictyol, carvacrol, thymol, rosmarinic, caffeic, *p*-coumaric, protocatechuic acid

A significant increase in antioxidants of 15-20% is possible by increasing consumption of Herbs, Spices, fruits and vegetables, particularly those high in ORAC values.

Increasing the amount of Phytonutrient rich foods in our diet can boost antioxidant activity and our immune health.They are best consumed through natural foods.

It is well said by Hippocrates, *"Let Food Be Thy Medicine and Medicine Be Thy Food".*

This is felt more relevant and apt in current pandemic where all natural foods including Herbs, Spices and Condiments have gained more importance for building immunity.

In this modern world with so much inventions in medical field and advancement of technology, natural foods, Herbs and Spices have shown their superiority. Our kitchen spices is the biggest pharmacy for the whole family. Spices are the heart and soul of Indian cuisine. Every kitchen shelf in India has different varieties of spices and herbs.

In various studies it is found that spices can potentially be used as ameliorative or preventive agents for some health issues. The World Health Organisation (WHO) and Ministry of Ayush, GoI have also strongly recommend Spices and Herbs as best immunity booster.

References

1. Allwyn Sundar Raj A., Aaron S., Seinenbalg S.S., Tiroutchelvamaa D., Ranganathan T.V. Review on recent trends in isolation of antioxidants from spices and its biological effects of essential oils. *J. Eng. Res. Appl.* 2014; 4: 75–84. [Google Scholar]
2. Asha Devi S., Umasanker M.E., Babu S. A comparative study of antioxidant properties in common Indian spices. *Int. Res. J. Pharm.* 2012; 3: 465–468. [Google Scholar]
3. Bhattacharjee S., Sengupta A. Spices in cancer prevention—An overview. *Internet J. Nutr. Wellness.* 2008; 7: 1–16. [Google Scholar]
4. D. Shoeman and B.C.Fielding, "Coronavirus envelope protein :current knowledge", *Virology Journal,* Vol. 16, No. 1, p. 69, 2019.
5. D. P. Jones, "Redefining oxidative stress," Antioxidants & Redox Signaling, Vol. 8, No. 9–10, pp. 1865–1879, 2006.
6. G. N. Kim and H. D. Jang, "Protective mechanism of quercetin and rutin using glutathione metabolism on H_2O_2- induced oxidative stress in HepG2 cells," *Annals of the New York Academy of Sciences,* Vol. 1171, No. 1, pp. 530–537, 2009.
7. H. Sies, "Oxidative stress: a concept in redox biology and medicine," *Redox Biology,* Vol. 4, pp. 180–183, 2015.
8. Kaefer C.M., Milner J.A. The role of herbs and spices in cancer prevention. *J. Nutr. Biochem.* 2008;19:347–354. doi: 10.1016/j.jnutbio.2007.11.003. [PMC free article] [PubMed] [CrossRef] [Google Scholar]
9. L. E. Gralinski and R. S. Baric, "Molecular pathology of emerging coronavirus infections," *The Journal of Pathology,* Vol. 235, No. 2, pp. 185–195, 2015.

10. S. Luo, X. Zhang, and H. Xu, "Don't overlook digestive symptoms in patients with 2019 novel coronavirus disease (COVID-19)," *Clinical Gastroenterology and Hepatology*, Vol. 18, No. 7, pp. 1636-1637, 2020.
11. S. Wu, Y. Zhang, F. Ren *et al.*, "Structure–affinity relationship of the interaction between phenolic acids and their derivatives and β-lactoglobulin and effect on antioxidant activity," *Food Chemistry*, Vol. 245, pp. 613-619, 2018.
12. Z. Zhou, N. Zhao, Y. Shu, S. Han, B. Chen, and X. Shu, "Effect of gastrointestinal symptoms in patients with COVID-19," *Gastroenterology*, Vol. 158, No. 8, pp. 2294–2297, 2020.
13. Z. Zhang, L. Rong, and Y.-P. Li, "Flaviviridae viruses and oxidative stress: implications for viral pathogenesis," Oxidative Medicine and Cellular Longevity, Vol. 2019, Article ID 1409582, 17 pages, 2019.
14. www.oracvalues.com
15. www.medicalnewstoday.com/articles/320721#canthe immune system be booster
16. www.nccih.nih.gov./health/antioxidants in depth
17. https://pubmed.ncbi.nim.nih.gov/32283152
18. https://pubmed.ncbi.nim.nih.gov/32438473
19. https://pubmed.ncbi.nim.nih.gov/pmc/articles/pmc6723551
20. https://pubmed.ncbi.nim.nih.gov/pmc/articles/pmc7280664/pdf/EJI-999911
21. https://pubmed.ncbi.nim.nih.gov/pmc/articles/pmc7187672

2

Impact of Covid-19 on Infant and Young Child Feeding Practices in India

Dr Rachana Srivastava, Dr Poonam Khanna, and Savitesh Kushwaha

Consistent surge in count of covid victims along with the actions to curb its spread has influenced: sources of income, availability and accessibility of food items and access to health and nutrition services like, antenatal and post-natal counselling, celebration of village health and nutrition days (VHND), early childhood care, education, growth monitoring and social safety nets, leading to health and nutritional status of countless people at stake. Most vulnerable are the infants and young children as they depend on others for access and consumption and have lower capacity to respond to the risks. Decline in early initiation and exclusive breastfeeding rates due to inadequate provision of routine healthcare services amid COVID-19 has already been reported. Slashed food availability at household level, coupled with multiple demands on parents due to lockdowns, has made minimum dietary diversity for young children a remote goal. Optimum infant and young child feeding practices are imperative for development of a healthy child, failure to which leads to poor health, compromised growth and cognitive development and mortality. This chapter deals with the challenges to infant and young child feeding practices created during this pandemic and evidences/ recommendations which can be converted into general practices nationwide, for positive outcomes.

It is well established that appropriate infant and young child feeding practices are imperative for development of a healthy child, failure to which leads to poor health, compromised growth and cognitive development and eventually mortality. Bettering infant and young child feeding (IYCF) practices can restore longevity, growth, and development of children with equity. Adequate and timely, infant and young child feeding (IYCF) practices can slash childhood infections (diarrhoea and pneumonia) and provide a strong foundation for the optimal growth and development of the child. Recognising the importance of nutrition in the first two years, age-appropriate infant and young child feeding (IYCF) interventions are being promoted worldwide.

Before pandemic only 41.6% infants were breastfed within 60 minutes of birth, 54.9% were exclusively breastfed for six months and 11.6% children aged 6-23 months were getting an adequate diet in India.[1,2] Covid-19 has emerged not only as a health catastrophe but as a social and economic risk, creating enormously challenging circumstances. Evidences suggest that children are marginally prone to Covid-19 but they were punched hardest as far as the food, nutrition and health security is concerned.[3]

World Food Programme predicts that the number of people facing adversity from acute food insecurity will be two-fold by the end of this year that is 270 million from 135 million. The count of moderately and severely wasted children in India could raise from about 23 million (before the commencement of the pandemic) to further 26 million.[4] Dearth of crucial nutrition services, disordered supply chains and soared food prices has added to household poverty and food insecurity, deteriorating the diet quality of children. Outcomes of the pandemic are instigating more damage to children than the disease itself.[5]

Constricted household incomes and rationing of vitamins and mineral rich foods due to supply interruptions in delivery chain due to pandemic is devastating for the world's most defenceless population, the children. Undernourishment in initial stages of life results in irreparable damages through the lifecycle. A deficient diet doesn't only delay neurocognitive maturity and educational achievement, it also diminishes working capacity and earnings in adulthood and enhances the risk of chronic disease and premature death. These difficulties resonate beyond individuals and hampers the potential of their societies too.[6]

The lockdown levied to curb the proliferation of COVID-19, disturbed the key service delivery and following that the strategic platform for delivery of core nutrition-specific interventions facilities, the Anganwadi centres were closed. As Accredited Social Health Activists (ASHAs), and ANMs were involved in COVID-19 duties of contact tracing and community awareness generation, they did not had time for their essential duties of supplementary nutrition delivery, nutrition counselling, early childhood care and growth monitoring etc. Also, upsurge in migrant exodus (5-30 million), affected the delivery of specific health and nutrition interventions.[7,8]

Optimal Infant and Young Child Feeding Practices

Optimal breastfeeding and complementary feeding practices can avert twenty percent of mortalities in children under five years of age. Risk of ailments like diarrhoea and pneumonia, (primary causes of mortality among children below five years) reduces if infants are exclusively breastfed for 6 months. Early initiation of breastfeeding, within the first hour of life, is identified as significant intervention for infant survival.[9] Infant and young child feeding practices are a set of guiding principles and technical recommendations for infants and children under two years of age. IYCF guidelines are shared in Table 1.[10, 11]

Table 1: Infant and young child feeding (IYCF) guidelines in India

	IYCF guidelines	*Details*
1.	Timely Initiation of breastfeeding	Immediately after birth, preferably within one hour.
2.	Exclusive breastfeeding for 6 months	180 days (no other foods or fluids, not even water; but allows infant to receive ORS, drops, syrups of vitamins, minerals and medicines when required)
3.	Timely initiation of complementary feeding	Solid, semisolid or soft foods after the age of six months i.e. 180 days.
4.	Breastfeeding for 2 years or till baby feeds	Continued breastfeeding for 2 years or beyond
5.	Age-appropriate complementary feeding for children 6-23 months, while continuing breastfeeding	Timely, adequate and safe food should be provided to children
	I) Minimum dietary diversity	Children should receive food from 4 or more food groups: (1) Grains, roots and tubers, legumes and nuts; (2) dairy products; (3) flesh foods (meat fish, poultry); (4) eggs, (5) vitamin A rich fruits and vegetables; (6) other fruits and vegetables

(Contd...)

	II) Minimum meal frequency	Children should be fed for a minimum number of times 2 times for breasted infants 6-8 months; 3 times for breastfed children 9-23 months; 4 times for non-breastfed children 6-23 months
6.	Active feeding for Children during and after illness	Feeding during sickness is important for recovery and for prevention of undernutrition.
7.	Consumption of iron rich foods	Children should receive iron rich or iron fortified food to curb anemia, (if an iron supplement is to be given, it is best provided after meals)

Interventions for promoting and supporting Infant and Young Child Feeding Practices in India

Government of India has launched many health and nutritional programmes and policies to support adequate and timely infant and young child feeding practices. The launch of these schemes has led to a re-prioritisation of nutrition outcomes, with clear targets being laid out to be achieved. Table 2 covers various programmes and schemes which support IYCF practices in India.

Table 2: Programmes and schemes supporting IYCF practices in India

	Schemes	*Features*
1.	Integrated Child Development Services (ICDS)	Provides basic education, health, and nutrition services for early childhood development and counselling for correct IYCF Via Anganwadi workers (AWWs)
2.	Mid-day meal	One hot cooked mid-day meal containing energy and protein, on each school day (at least 200 days in a year).
3.	National Health Mission (NHM)	Focus on enhancing maternal and child health ANMs and ASHAs reinforce appropriate IYCF practices during home visits and outreach activities.
4.	Poshan Abhiyaan	Aims to holistically diminish the malnutrition incidence in India by 2022 using technology including the ICDS Common Application System (ICDS-CAS) a real-time monitoring system and job aid convergence; capacity building; and behaviour change communication.

(Contd...)

5.	Pradhan Mantri Matritva Vandana Yojana (PMMVY)	A maternity benefit scheme designed to compensate wage loss of women and promoting health and nutrition seeking behaviour
6.	Janani suraksha yojna	Encourage Infant and Young Child Feeding practices through messages, counselling and advice during healthcare service delivery and informal communication with the beneficiaries

Challenges encountered in executing schemes:

- Lack of coverage and access, and household aspirations to seek private services, due to perception that government services are of poorer quality.
- Inequitable access and exclusion, quality and quantity of food supplements remains low in several states.
- High vacancies for doctors and specialists in National Health Mission.
- Low awareness, cumbersome procedures, and delayed payments result in women not receiving their entitlements.[12]

Covid-19 and Breastfeeding

Supporting the breastfeeding rates is the superlative intervention in improving the health of a population. Breastfeeding encourages proximity and bonding and thus promotes mental health of both mother and baby and reduces health inequalities too.[13]

Till date there is no confirmation of COVID-19 virus transmittal of from mother to infant in-utero or through breast milk. WHO and UNICEF suggest that mothers who are suspected, probable, or confirmed case of COVID-19 should follow standard infant feeding practices with the application of all precautions of prevention and control of infections. It includes keeping mothers and infants together (rooming-in), continuous and prolonged skin-to-skin contact immediately after birth, introduction of breastfeeding within one hour of birth, and exclusive breastfeeding. Mothers should mandatorily take Infection Prevention and Control (IPC) precautions, including using medical mask, hand washing and cleaning of frequently touched surfaces.[14]

A study, conducted by BPNI (Breastfeeding Promotion Network of India) revealed important knowledge and practices gaps among the breastfeeding counsellors in India. There is a need of on-going updating and orientation of these trained professionals with the technical information about the safety and necessity of breastfeeding by the Covid-19 positive mothers. Also, the pregnant and lactating women should be helped with correct information about breastfeeding in Covid-19 situation in local language and using easy to understand print and electronic instruments to address the anxiety about practicing breastfeeding in view of Covid-19 pandemic.[15]

Covid-19 and lockdown has disrupted routine healthcare system and aggravated the situation of nutrition insecurity in pregnant and lactating mothers of disadvantaged groups, due to lack of antenatal and postnatal counselling sessions and insufficiency of support / handholding on breastfeeding, colostrum feeding procedure from healthcare workers like auxiliary nurse midwife (ANM) and Anganwadi workers (AWW) as they were deputed for COVID-19 duty. A drop in incidence of breastfeeding is anticipated owing to unwillingness of women to use healthcare system, restraints in health services delivery and utilisation, and dearth of skilled health workers which can eventually lead to partial addressal of ante-natal and post-natal care, and facility and community-based lactation support and counselling.[16]

Breastfeeding is found to be effective against many infectious diseases. Therefore, mothers should maintain utmost hygiene and should wash her hands while feeding or expressing breast milk with a breast pump to avoid spreading the virus to the baby, also ensure cleaning of pump or bottle parts before and after each use. A nutritious and balanced diet along with psychological assessment and support, should be given to lactating mothers so as to improve their health. Selections made in these difficult times should be evidence-based. Prolonging/ continuing breastfeeding is an evidence-based practice, for protecting the health of new borns and is now more important than ever, to ensure that the child receives the best start of his/her life.[17]

Covid-19 and Complementary Feeding and Young Child Feeding Practices

Breastfeeding must be complemented with safe and nutritionally adequate, solid, semi-solid and soft age-appropriate foods from six months of life. This complementary feeding period from 6 to 24 months is an important part of the first thousand days of life. It has been estimated that about 100,000 deaths in children younger than five years due to malnutrition could be prevented each year if complementary feeding was appropriate. But during the pandemic, mothers and caregivers face various challenges to providing appropriate feeds to their young ones.[18]

More than 60 million children are aided by the midday meal scheme in anganwadi centres, in India, which contributes a significant part of their daily dietary intake. These meals are vital both for child nourishment and mental development. Moreover, many families use creche services of anganwadis to take care of their children when they are away for work, as most of the anganwadi centres were not operational during the pandemic, taking up employment was problematic for parents with young children. Dry rations distribution or cash transfers have been initiated in many states from July but hot cooked meals are still a distant dream. Hot cooked meals are meant to ensure that the food is consumed by the child, and is not shared among family members. Importance of missed nutrition cannot be emphasised enough by saying that this budding generation is endangered of losing its potential and economic contributions to nation's future and for above 200 million Indian children, the brunt of cut down nutrition will persist all through their lifetime.[19]

Albeit of precautionary actions taken by government to safeguard adversity of the lockdown on the harvesting, transporting, procurement and storage of the food grains, inevitable breaches in the infrastructure, have raised the cost of vegetables, fruits and poultry enormously in several localities. The quality of complementary feeds is mostly enriched by addition of extra ghee, oil, sugar, jaggery and addition of fruits, vegetables, egg and poultry. Inspite of low family income, many families arrange these items specifically for infants, which has been difficult in present times. Lockdown and limited availability of fresh foods has resulted in amplified usage of packed, ready to cook, highly processed nutrient deficient calorie rich food items. Complementary feeds thus lack the minimum meal diversity and hence adequacy.[20]

With trivial improvement in instigating food security allowance, or dry rations, and existing poor IYCF practices, the other challenges surfaced during this crisis are: fallacies about breastfeeding, food insecurity obstructing the availability of nutritious food, contending household requirements, mental trauma that affects childcare practices and interruption in utilisation of standard nutrition services. Those young ones whose first 1000 days of life intersect with this contagion are especially jeopardised.[21]

Covid-19 and Malnutrition

Developmental epigenetic researches corroborate that the consequences of under nutrition and deprivation on neurocognitive and brain development of the child are lasting and salvaging from them is often unattainable, and is partially likely, only when unfavourable home and societal conditions improve. A current study from Gambia suggested that deprived maternal nutrition during conception induced lasting changes in their baby's DNA methylation, permanently altering the function of important genes. Hence, this pandemic can have brutal ramifications on undernourished children as they are at an ever-high risk of death and poor growth, development and learning.

As per projections, UNICEF presages that Covid-19 contributed to global food scarcity and intrusion in health system which increased the number of wasted children under the age of five years by a distressing 6.7 million in the initial year of the pandemic. A 4.3 percent upsurge in incidence of wasting among children below the age of five in low and middle-income countries (LMIC) was also forecasted by the Lancet analysis. Wasting or less weight for age is a lethal condition, which leads to thinness in children, imperils them of dying, poor growth, and inadequate development and learning. Wasted children become 3 to 12 times more vulnerable to death than children with a healthy body weight.[22]

The expected economic depression and unemployment will contribute to rise in food insecure families and thus the probability of a child being severely stunted, severely underweight or severely wasted belonging to such families is increased.[23]

Acute and severe wasting, or thinness, is referred as Severe Acute Malnutrition (SAM). SAM children are more vulnerable to infections and mortality risk is eight-fold higher among them as compared to well-nourished children. Covid-19 will lead to augmented wasting incidences in SAM children despite of food aids, safety net programmes, etc, as countless people have lost their income which in turn affects household food inaccessibility as well as quantity and quality of diet.

Challenges

This pandemic has detrimental effects on growth and development of children, especially those who were already in the throes of malnutrition and poverty. The challenges in achieving appropriate infant and young child feeding during this pandemic were:

- Shutting of anganwadi centres and schools which led to interruptions in nutrition service delivery across India.
- Disruption in the supply chain logistics in keeping the services running.

- Non-availability of food in local market due to panic purchases of food break the supply chain and also caused localised price hikes affecting the children in lower socioeconomic strata.
- Transport bans and border closures between states altered the local availability and price of the food despite of government's efforts to ensure availability of essential commodities.[24]
- Job cuts pushed the weaker sections into acute poverty and limited their ability to access nutritious food.
- Closure of factories and businesses caused mass exodus of the workers and daily wagers along with their families. Providing to the nutritional needs of these children on the move was also a challenge.[25]

Applied Interventions

Long term nutrition security is endangered and its health and economic impacts will be extensive and precarious for the children across the nation due to provisional suspension of mid-day meals and supplementary nutrition programmes.[26] Therefore, it is of utmost value to retain crucial maternal and child health and nutrition facilities streaming so that antenatal care can be attended by mothers for a healthy pregnancy; infants are delivered securely with skilful birth attendants; infants and young children are vaccinated, shielded and treated for diseases and infections, obtain micronutrient supplements as required, and are breastfed and complementary fed timely and safely and counselling should also be delivered about nutritious foods and healthy diets to caregivers. Robust evidences exist and support that these strategies are extremely effective in averting under nutrition if implemented well.[27]

- The availability of food for child nutrition during this crisis, households received food subsidies and cash transfers has been ensured.
- The food systems were strengthened during pandemic and home delivery of supplementary nutrition was ensured to cater adequate nutrition for women and children.

Way ahead

COVID-19 has reinforced the unpreparedness of the world to protect its citizens against starvation and uncertainties of food, nutrition and health in global crisis situations. Impending wellbeing of the world now depends on reconfiguring the current ineffective food, nutrition, health and social protection structures to guarantee food security for all.[28]

Social safety nets

Targeted social safety net programmes, payment deferrals, or tax breaks as well as suitable cash-support programs for the most vulnerable are required. Targeting the most marginalised households in rural populations and urban slums could be achieved through deploying community health workers and supporting women and community members.

Relief programmes

Relief programmes are required to improve intra household resources and food distribution for mothers and young children and to shield them from domestic violence and psychosocial stress, which could otherwise will have severe negative effects on children.[29]

Eat local

Locally available fresh vegetables and fruits from the homestead or nutrition gardens are a major, sustainable and affordable way of ensuring availability of healthy food, balanced diet, dietary diversity, nutrition and micronutrients. Nutrition gardens tend to improve the household consumption of nutritious food, promote dietary diversity and increase the quantity of fruits and vegetables consumed in the household.[30] Focus should also be paid in procuring locally grown horticultural crops to households under the MDM and ICDS umbrella for enhancing nutrient density and diet diversity for children. This can also be an instrument in offering provisional relief to farmers through local procurement.[31]

Scaling up nutrition services

A prompt and judicious evaluation of the outreach and effectiveness of the prevailing nutrition interventions and programmes is imperative and a well-planned approach that assumes that all necessary measures, including the Poshan Abhiyan, can positively influence children's nutrition and their well-being.[32,33] School feeding and other food assistance programmes should be resumed for delivering meals to quarantined families with young children, pregnant and lactating women i.e. to assist those who are at immediate risk of food shortages.[34]

Swachh bharat Surakshit bharat

Community-led sanitation programmes could be key to ensuring healthy household environments and reducing undernutrition. Hand hygiene for both caregivers and infants needs to be stressed. The practice of providing a separate plate/katori/spoon/glass to each child will also decrease disease transmission.

Breastfeeding- A boon

The protective effect of breastfeeding is particularly strong against infectious diseases. Breastfeeding protects against illnesses and death in the post-neonatal period, throughout infancy and childhood. For this, breastfeeding should be initiated within the first hour of birth. Exclusive breastfeeding should continue for six months with timely introduction of adequate, safe and properly fed complementary foods at age six months, while continuing breastfeeding up to two years of age or beyond.[35,36]

Additionally, several COVID-19 response measures such as contact tracing and self-isolation could also be exploited for nutrition protection. Global health and improvements in undernutrition will require governments, donors, and development partners to restrategise and reprioritise investments for the COVID-19 era, and will necessitate data-driven decision making, political will and commitment, and international unity. These steps if implemented now can prevent the pandemic from further undermining child nutrition.

References

1. India (IND) -Demographics, Health & Infant Mortality -UNICEF DATA. Available at https://data.unicef.org. Accesses on May 3, 2020.
2. National Family Health Survey-Fact sheet. Available at http://rchiips.org. Accesses on May 3, 2020.
3. Ghosh, R, Dubey, MJ, Chatterjee, S, Dubey, S. Impact of Covid-19 on children: special focus on the psychosocial aspect. Minerva Pediatr 2020; 72: 226-35. dOi: 10.23736/S0026-4946.20.05887-9.
4. https://poshan.outlookindia.com/story/poshan-news-covid-19-and-the-irreversible-marks-undernutrition-will-leave-in-its-wake/366864.
5. https://indianexpress.com/article/parenting/health-fitness/additional-6-7-million-children-under-5-could-suffer-from-wasting-due-to-covid-19-unicef-6527619.
6. Supporting children's nutrition during the COVID-19 pandemic. Available at https://www.unicef.org.Accessed on 15 May 2020.
7. Accountability Initiative. 2020. Inside Districts. Accountability Initiative, Centre for Policy Research. Available online at: https://www.insidedistricts.com/.
8. Chishti, S. June 2020. Explained: How many migrant workers displaced? A range of estimates. Indian Express. Available online at: https://indianexpress.com/article/explained/coronavirus-how-many-migrant-workers-displaced-a-rangeof-estimates-6447840/.

9. https://timesofindia.indiatimes.com/blogs/the-interviews-blog/breastfeeding-and-complementary-feeding-practices-together-can-prevent-almost-20-of-deaths-in-children-under-five-years.
10. http://www.nrhmorissa.gov.in/writereaddata/Upload/Documents/Guideline%20-%20IYCF.pdf
11. https://www.ennonline.net/attachments/987/final-iycf-guide-iycf-practices.pdf
12. https://accountabilityindia.in/wp-content/uploads/2020/12/Nutrition-Brief_.pdf
13. World Health Organisation. (2020). Breastfeeding and COVID-19: scientific brief, 23June 2020. World Health Organisation.
14. https://apps.who.int/iris/handle/10665/332639
15. https://www.bpni.org/wp-content/uploads/2020/11/Covid-19-and-Breastfeeding-a-quantitative-study.pdf
16. UNICEF(2020) - Infant & young child feeding in the context of Covid-19; Brief No. 2 (v1); March 30th, 2020. https://www.unicef.org/media/68281/file/IYCF-Programming-COVID19-Brief.pdf
17. https://www.downtoearth.org.in/blog/health/breastfeeding-in-times-of-covid-19-will-newborns-miss-out-on-vital-nutrition-72668
18. https://poshan.outlookindia.com/story/poshan-news-breastfeeding-during-a-pandemic/350248
19. WHO (2020). Clinical management of Covid –19, Interim guidance, 27th May, 2020. https://www.who.int/publications/i/item/clinical-management-of-covid-19
20. https://indianexpress.com/article/parenting/health-fitness/additional-6-7-million-children-under-5-could-suffer-from-wasting-due-to-covid-19-unicef-6527619/
21. Varghese, A., Agarwal, M., 2020. Safeguarding nutritional opportunities of first 1000 days of life during a pandemic: infant and young children feeding practices in the context of COVID-19 in India. International Journal of Community Medicine and Public Health 7, 2836. doi:10.18203/2394-6040.ijcmph20203023.
22. Alvi, M., & Gupta, M. (2020). Learning in times of lockdown: how Covid-19 is affecting education and food security in India. *Food security*, 1–4. Advance online publication. https://doi.org/10.1007/s12571-020-01065-4.
23. https://poshan.outlookindia.com/story/poshan-news-covid-19-and-the-irreversible-marks-undernutrition-will-leave-in-its-wake/366864.
24. Economic Times Online. Delhi schools closed: All primary schools shut as corona virus spreads. The Economic Times. [Newspaper on the internet]. 2020. Available from: https://m.economictimes.com/news/politics-andnation/coronavirus-in-india-all-primary-schools-in-delhito-be-shut-till-march-31/articleshow/74493367.cms
25. Acharya, R. July 2020. Reduced Food and Diet Quality, and Need for Nutrition Services During Covid-19: Findings from Surveys in Bihar and Uttar Pradesh. International Food Policy Research Institute South Asia. Available online at: https://southasia.ifpri.info/2020/07/09/15081/.https://www.ifpri.org/blog/how-indias-agrifood-supply-chains-fared-during-covid-19-lockdown-farm-fork
26. https://scroll.in/article/973716/as-indias-children-miss-midday-meals-due-to-school-closures-how-can-adequate-nutrition-be-ensured

27. https://health.economictimes.indiatimes.com/news/industry/we-will-witness-a-surge-in-covid-19-generation-of-malnourished-children-dr-rajan-sankar-director-nutrition-tata-trusts/79617036
28. https://poshan.outlookindia.com/story/poshan-news-nutrition-in-the-context-of-the-covid-19-pandemic-in-india/354455
29. Singh, S, Fernandes, M. Home-grown school feeding: Promoting local production systems diversification through nutrition sensitive agriculture. Food Security. 2018; 10(1):111–119. doi: 10.1007/s12571-017-0760-5
30. https://www.downtoearth.org.in/blog/health/covid-19-role-of-nutrition-gardens-in-ensuring-nutrition-for-children-72777
31. https://indianexpress.com/article/opinion/columns/the-kids-are-not-alright-2-7110543/
32. Avula, R, Kaur, S, and Menon, P. 2020. Protecting India's Health and Nutrition Programs Amidst Covid-19 Pandemic. International Food Policy Research Institute South Asia. Available online at: https://southasia.ifpri.info/2020/05/20/ protecting-indias-health-and-nutrition-programs-amidst-covid-19-pandemic
33. Paina, L., and Peters. D.H. (2012). Understanding pathways for scaling up health services through the lens of complex adaptive systems. Health Policy Plan. 27(5):365373. doi:10.1093/heapol/czr054
34. https://poshan.outlookindia.com/story/poshan-news-breastfeeding-during-a-pandemic/350248
35. Upadhyay, MK, Patra, S, Khan, AM. Ensuring availability of food for child nutrition amidst the COVID–19 pandemic: Challenges and Way forward. Indian J Comm Health. 2020;32(2-Special Issue): 251-254.
36. Nadia Akseer, Goutham Kandru, Emily C Keats, Zulfiqar A Bhutta. COVID-19 pandemic and mitigation strategies: implications for maternal and child health and nutrition, *The American Journal of Clinical Nutrition*, Volume 112, Issue 2, August 2020, Pages 251–256, https://doi.org/10.1093/ajcn/nqaa171.

3

Ayurvedic Nutritional and Immunity Boosting Perspective of *Ahara* (Diet) in Pre-Conception and Pregnancy during COVID Era

Dr Anuradha Roy

"The food is the vital force of life. All living beings are dependent on food for complexion, cheerfulness, good voice, happiness, contentment, corpulence, strength, intellect and long live. All worldly (for livelihood), vedic (for heavenly abode) and activities for liberation depend on food.*" (Caraka Samhita. Sutra Sthana. 27/Verse no. 349-351)*

Every person depends on food especially for living and for living healthy one should take food in proper quantity. Quantity depends on the power of digestion (*agnibala*). According to Ayurveda, measured proper quantity food is that which gets easily digested in time without disturbing the normalcy of *doshas* (bodily humours) and *agni* (digestive fires). The food item as red *sali* (rice variety), *mudga* (green gram), *saindhava* (rock salt), *jivanti* (L reticukat as leafy vegetable), *amalaki* (fruit), cow's milk and ghee, sesame oil, ginger, grapes etc are naturally wholesome to all individuals. The diet which are light in nature due to predominance of *vayu* and *agnimahabhuta* (basic elements), stimulates digestion and hence even though taken up to the saturation point produces little derangement. On the other hand, diets heavy in digestion are predominant of *prthvi* and *jalamahabhuta* which are not digestive stimulant, when taken up to the saturation point, produces considerable derangement. For maintenance of health the concept of *pathya* (wholesome) and *apathya* (un-wholesome) is the key. *Pathya* is that which is not harmful to the *patha* (macro and micro channels of the body) and is according to liking. Therefore, only the use of wholesome food promotes the growth of a person and that of unwholesome one is the cause of disorders.

Ayurveda narrates much of pre-conception as the best period to groom the physical and mental faculties of the upcoming progeny by prescribing specified dietary intake. Pregnancy is a phase which is to be taken care of in all aspect specially diet. So the regular diet with little modifications, beneficial for both mother and intrauterine fetus to be considered. A woman should be concerned towards the quality of food rather than the type and quantity of food. Ayurveda also provides personalised recommendations about which foods to eat and avoid based on one's *prakriti* (body constitution), which is determined by predominance of *dosha* (body humors).

During this current pandemic COVID-19, which is caused by severe acute respiratory syndrome coronavirus-2 (SARSCoV2) spreading rapidly across the globe possesses a major health concern. Compared to available measures in conventional system, in Ayurveda, majority of interventions are provided through immune-boosting measures. Pregnancy is a state of immunological change, thus considered under vulnerable group. So, it is highly recommended to provide diet which is nutritional and possessing quantified immunity boosting herbs as a component to such women rather than only healthy diet. Ayurveda emphasises on *Ahara* with special reference to pre-conception and pregnancy and its holistic management.

Pre-Conception Diet

Pre-conception care is defined as the provision of biomedical, behavioural and social health interventions to a women or a couple before conception. Ayurveda helps the couple planning for parenthood for both physical and mental health prepared for *Shreyasipraja* (best progeny in quality). *Ahara* plays a very important role before and during pregnancy as it decides the future health of the fetus to be born. According to Ayurveda just after menstruation on 4th day onwards the couple after being purified by use of oleation, sudatory measures, *vamana* (emasis), *virechana* (purgation) and following proper dietetics should use specific diet for man and woman to get a *prasasthagarbha* (best progeny in quality). For man should use the *ghrita* and milk medicated with the drugs of *madhuravarga* (sweet or anabolic drugs). *Ghrita* is *sheetavirya* having *vata-pitta* pacifying properties and milk with *madhuravarga* drugs have *rasayana* properties all beneficial for *sukra* and *ojas*. All these *Ahara* are advised with a view to better functioning of *shukra* which helps in attaining conception with optimum quality. In female, *taila* (oil) and *masa* (a type of kidney bean) are advised to be consumed. *Taila* promotes strength (*balya*) and helps in *Garbhashaya Vishodhana* (cleanses reproductive tract). *Tila taila* help the female for maintaining the reproductive capacity by enhancing the healthy conception. Also *masa* is *vatahara*, *madhura rasa*, *ushnavirya* and *snigdha* property. All these diets are rich source of folic acid, proteins, and fibers and are antioxidant; it helps to reduce oxidative stress, thus increases healthy fertility.

In the form of *rasayana- Phalaghreeta* or *mahakalyanaghrita* are beneficial.

For all pre-conception and during pregnancy *ritucharya* (seasonal dietetic regimen) in terms of *Ahara* can be followed as below:

Hemanta Ritu and Sisira Ritu (Winter seasons)	***Vasanta Ritu (Spring season)***	***Grishma Ritu (Summer season)***
• Sweet, sour and salt taste predominant food items • Unctuous meat soup • Food preparation with jaggery • Black gram • Food items prepared with sugarcane • Food items prepared with milk • Freshly harvested rice • Til Taila • Hot water	• Light food items • Old barley • Wheat • Honey • Sweet mango juice • Dry ginger or honey with boiled water • Green gram soup	• Thin gruels prepared with cornflour and sugar • Sali rice with mutton soup • Rasala (curds churned without any water and mixed with sugar, pepper, dry ginger) • Khandava (prepared with sour and sweet fruits) • Pancasara (a type of mantha prepared with draksha, kharjura, madhuka, kashmarya and parushaka) • Buffalo milk with sugar

***Varsha Ritu* (Rainy season)**	***Sarad Ritu* (Autumn season)**
• Old barley, wheat and Sali rice along with meat soup • Sour and salt predominant food • Boiled and cool water	• Bitter, sweet, astringent taste predominant food items • Sali rice • Green gram • Sugar • Amla • Honey • Mutton soup • Milk

Garbhakara Ahara (Fertility enhancing)

- Pulses- *moog dal, urad daal.*
- Whole grains.
- Fresh fruits and vegetables.
- Spices- *ajwain* (bishop's weed), cumin (which purifies the uterus in women), turmeric (to improve the interaction between hormones and targeted tissues), black cumin, fennel, cinnamon, and cardamom.
- Pomegranate- help in thickening the uterine lining, which reduces the chances of pregnancy loss.
- Garlic- known for improving fertility. 4 to 5 cloves of garlic to be chewed. Drink a glass of warm milk after chewing the garlic cloves. This may be followed specially during winters.
- Nutmeg also enhance fertility can be taken equal amounts of nutmeg powder and sugar powder (approximately 3 grams each) with one cup milk.
- Tulsi- three to four leaves can be chewed daily, followed by a glass of milk to improve fertility.
- Cinnamon- helps in better functioning of ovaries. A teaspoon of cinnamon powder in a cup of warm water and drink this tea for a few months, or can sprinkle it on top of any meals.
- Rock Salt- has many essential minerals in it like calcium, magnesium, potassium and iron. Help in enhancing fertility.
- Vitamin D- lack of Vitamin D may lead to infertility and even abortion, is very important to strengthen bones, teeth and muscles, and improves calcium absorption. The best way is early morning sunlight for 10 minutes and eats vitamin D-rich foods such as egg yolk and cheese.

Garbhini Ahara (pregnancy diet)

Pregnancy is one of the most beautiful journey of a woman life, a demanding phase both physically and psychologically. This demand can be modified by *Ahara* (food).The diet during pregnancy has to be rich in calories, proteins, vitamins and minerals and should be well balanced. Thus, needs a regimen which provides extra energy and nutrient support to produce a positive healthy pregnancy outcome. Ayurveda has very vividly described the monthwise dietary regime for healthy mother and the fetus. Thus, any woman desirous of eventless pregnancy and healthy good looking child should indulge in congenial diet always. Pregnant women should always be given *jivaniya* and *brimhaniya* (anabolic diet). She should always use butter, milk and ghee in her diet. One should consume after considering *matra* (quantity), *yoga* (combination), *desha* (geographical location), *kala* (time), *ritu* (season), *agni* (digestive fire), *swabhava* (inherent property), *samskara* (processing) etc.

Pregnancy period is divided in three trimesters. First trimester (1st to 3rd month), second trimester (4th to 6th month), and third trimester (7th to 9th month). So as the dietary planning goes month wise of pregnancy.

1st Trimester *Garbhini Ahara* (Pregnancy diet)

During the 1st trimester (first three months of pregnancy), as majority of the women have nausea and vomiting and cannot take a diet properly. Use of *madhura* (sweet), *sheeta* (cold) and *drava Ahara* (liquid diet) diet will prevent her from getting dehydrated and also supply proper nutrition to both mother and fetus. Also all the *madhura* groups of drugs are anabolic in nature and help maintaining the pregnancy. By taking milk, fetus get nourishment and stability.

Garbhini Ahara (Pregnancy diet) during first month

First month is a stage to stabilise thus when women have doubt of having pregnancy or confirmed her pregnancy she should take milk repeatedly in desired quantity. While taking any diet she should always consider her digestive fire and strength. Consideration for *pathya* (congenial) and *apathy* (non-congenial) *ahara* and always indulge in *pathya* (congenial) and *satmya* (favourable diet) *ahar* in the morning and evening. Pregnancy during first month needs extra nutrition for developing fetus and pregnant woman herself.

- *Madura* (sweet), *sheet* (cold), *drava ahara* (liquid diet) should be taken for the first three months.
- *Anupasamskritaksheera* (non-medicated milk) which is *sheeta* (cold) should be given repeatedly.
- Milk can also be medicated with some medicinal herbs as *Shaliparni (Desmodium* gangeticum *DC.), Palasha (Butea* monosperma*), Yasthimadhu (Glycyrrhiza* glabra Linn.*), Parushaka (Grewia* asiatica Linn.*)* and *Madhukapushpa (Diploknema* butyracea Roxb.*)* should be taken with butter and honey followed by milk.

- Water to be boiled with gold and silver and then given to drink once cooled. It is also considered to be auspicious.
- Administration of *swadu* (sweet), *sheeta* (cold), *drava ahara* (liquid diet) which are already *satmya* (favourable diet).

Garbhini Ahara (Pregnancy diet) during second month

During second month fetus attain the shape and sex is also differentiated. The pregnant lady needs a regimen which will prevent dehydration and supply nourishment. *Madura* drugs (sweet quality) are anabolic and help in maintenance of pregnancy.

- Milk medicated with *madhura* (sweet) drugs e.g. *Kakoli (Roscoraprcera*Wall.)
- All regimen advices in first month should be followed as such.

Garbhini Ahara (Pregnancy diet) during third month

Indriyas (sensory organs) and body parts develop simultaneously in fetus during this month. Here both mother and fetus needs regimen which supply adequate fluid and nutrition. Also the diet should be easily digestible and wholesome.

- Milk with honey and *ghrita* may be taken in a proper dose.
- *Krisara* (a recipe of rice and pulses) should be taken and is best.
- Regimen advices in first month should be followed as such.

  Shashti rice (a variety of rice) should be cooked in milk with added *madhura* (sweet), *sheeta* (cold) and *drava Ahara* (liquid diet).

2nd Trimester *Garbhini Ahara* (Pregnancy diet)

During second trimester of pregnancy as more body mass of the fetus is increased thus it is needed more have above mentioned diet. Hence provide such food stuff which is easily and quickly digestible items.

Garbhini Ahara (Pregnancy diet) during fourth month

Fetus gain stability also various body parts become more conspicuous during this month. Consciousness and heart develops. Woman feels more heaviness in the body due to stability of the fetus.

- Butter extracted from milk in measured quantity or milk with butter should be taken.
- Cooked *Shastika* rice (a variety of rice) with curd, dainty and pleasant food mixed with milk and butter and meat should be taken.

- Milk with butter should be given.

During this month fetus attain *sthiratva* (stability) as placenta is developed. From this month onwards the muscular tissue of the fetus grows sufficiently requiring more protein which is supplied by *mamsarasa* (meat soup) and dairy products (milk, ghee, curd).

Garbhini Ahara (Pregnancy diet) during fifth month

Accumulation of flesh and blood to the fetus is relatively more. *Mana* is enlightened in this month. Hence needs a regimen which helps in the mental development of the fetus. During this month the woman becomes emaciated due to lack of nourishment of maternal *dhatus* as *rasa* is driven to nourish more and more flesh and blood to fetus.

- *Ghrita* prepared from butter extracted from milk should be taken.
- Cooked *shastika* rice (a variety of rice) with milk and meat soup is to be taken.
- *Yavagu* (rice gruel)
- *Payasa* (Kheer)

Garbhini Ahara (Pregnancy diet) during sixth month

In pregnancy during this month fetus attain more *bala* (strength) and *varna* (complexion) than other months so mother suffers from loss of *bala* and *varna*. In this month enlightment of *buddhi* is more. Development of hair, nails, bones, tendons and quivering of fetus is more during this month.

- *Ghrita* prepared from milk medicated with the drugs of *madhura* group.
- *Ghrita* or *yavagu* (rice gruel) medicated with *gokshura* should be taken in desired quantity.
- Sweetened curd should be given.

During this month, as most of the women suffer from edema of feet etc, *gokshura* being a diuretic and rasayana will prevent water retention and its complication.

3rd Trimester *Garbhini Ahara* (Pregnancy diet)

3rd trimester is the last but most crucial period of pregnancy and below special diet is recommended.

Garbhini Ahara (Pregnancy diet) during seventh month

During this month the fetus attain full maturity, woman feels very exhausted. All the major and minor body parts are more conspicuous or are fully developed. The regimen during this month should contain drugs which are diuretic, anabolic, relieve emaciation and suppress *pitta* and *kapha*. During this month *Ghrita* medicated with *Prithakaparnyadi* group of drugs should be taken.

- *Ghrita khanda* (a sweet dish) should be given.

Garbhini Ahara (Pregnancy diet) during eighth month

During this month there are alternative states of excitement and depression in fetus and mother. This is explained nicely with the term *ojasanchara.*

- For clearing the long term constipated and retained feces and for *anulomana* (carminative) of *vayu*, the *asthapanavasti* should be given with the decoction of *badari* mixed with *bala, atibala, shatapushpa, patala*, milk, curd, mastu, oil, salt, *madanaphala*, honey and *ghrita.*
- It should be followed by the use of *anuvasanavasti* of oil medicated with milk and decoction of *madhura* group of drugs.
- Due to *anulomana* of *vayu*, the woman delivers without difficulty and remains free from complications.
- After this she should be given *snigdhayavagu* and *jangalamamsa rasa.*
- The body of woman thus treated becomes *snigdha*, she gains strength and delivers normally without any complications.
- Use of enema during the 8th month relieves constipation and provides base for uterine contractions.
- *Eneme* of oil medicated with *bala, atibala, shatapushpa* should be given followed by enema of sour substance like rock salt.
- *Yavagu* prepared with milk and mixed with *ghrita* should be taken.
- *Yavagu* prepared with milk and mixed with *ghrita* should be taken.

Garbhini Ahara (Pregnancy diet) during ninth month

Pregnancy during this month there is a state of full maturity, where vata needs to be regularised.

- *Asthapanavasti* (medicated *kashaya* rectal enema) for *anulomana* of *vata* (*vata* regulation).

- Use of *anulomanavasti* (medicated *sneha* rectal enema) with oil prepared with the drugs of *madhura* group or the same as used in eighth month is beneficial.
- *Yoni pichu* of oil should be given for lubrication of *garbhasthanamarga*; as it helps in relaxation of perineum and results in normal labour.
- *Anuvasanavasti* and *yoni picu* with *taila.*
- Meat soup with rice and *ghrita*
- *Bahusnehayavagu*
- *Anuvasanavasti*
- *Yoni picu* with *taila* daily
- *Snana* with *seta kashaya* of *vatagnapatra.*
- Different varieties of cereal should be given for 9th and 10th month.
- *Anuvasanataila* with *kadambamashataila* should be given.

Special concern during COVID era

During this COVID-19 outbreak, managing pre-conception and pregnancy becomes quite important and needs intelligent management as the women come under vulnerable group. Thus, prevention from getting infected or increasing body immunity against the virus is presently stressed upon. Though different steps for combating COVID-19 and prevent transmission of the virus are being practiced, but there is growing worldwide anxiety of being infected sooner or later by this virus. It is imperative to find a long-term solution to live in COVID era by adopting a holistic approach of Ayurveda to prevent or cure of physical, psychological, social and spiritual suffering. Ayurveda is a science of life, it teaches us to lead a happy and prosperous life with its basic principles even during this COVID crisis. In Ayurveda to achieve conception four essential factors are required- *Ritu* (normal menstrual cycle/ proper fertile period), *Kshetra* (healthy internal female reproductive organs), *Ambu* (good nutritional status of the female) and *Beeja* (healthy ovum in female and spermatozoa in male). Females have a great role as all four factors are related to her. Ayurveda gives prime importance to the preventive aspect and elaborates pre-conception and pregnancy diet for best quality progeny then and now even during pandemic.

AYUSH Guidelines:

- Eat freshly prepared warm food when hungry.

- Liquids – Instead of Tea, either of the following are advised Herbal tea prepared from ½ inch ginger + 2 Black pepper + ¼ cinnamon or lemon grass, *tulsi* leaves in 2 cups boiled water reduce it to 1 Cup and add honey 1 teaspoon.
- 1 cup hot cow's milk + dry Ginger powder/*Haridra* ½ teaspoon.
- Cereals – *Shalishashtika* (Old Rice) / *Laja*/ *Godhuma* (Wheat) / *Yava* (Barley).
- Pulses - *Mudga* (Phaseolus radiatus Linn), *Masur* (Lens culinaris Medic), *Kulattha* (Dolichos biflorus Linn.), *Chanaka*, *Moth*.
- Vegetables - *Vaartak* (Solanum melongena L), *Karkotak* (Momordica dioica Roxb. ex Willd.), *Shigru* (Moringa oleifera Lam), *Karvellaka* (Momordica charantia Linn), *Patola* (Tricosanthes dioica. Roxb), *Patha* (Cissampelosparieta Linn.), *Vaastuka* (Chenopodium album L.), *Jivanti* (Leptadenia reticulata (Retz.) Wight & Arn), *Tanduliyak* (Amaranthus spinosus L.), *Kakamachi* (Solanum nigrum Linn), *Guduchi* (Tinospora cordifolia. (Thunb.) Miers.)
- Fruits - *Draksha* (Vitis vinifera L.), *Kapittha* (Feronia limonia (Linn.)), *Dadima* (Punicagranatum Linn) can be taken.
- Condiments and spices: Cardamom/dry ginger/ black pepper/ long pepper/ garlic.

Rasayana for pregnant and lactating women

- *Phala Sarpis* - 10-12 gm in two divided doses with warm water.
- *Kalyanaka Ghrita* - 10-12 gm in two divided doses with warm water.
- *Ashwagandha Rasayana* - 10-12 gm twice daily with warm milk.
- *Soubhagya Shunti Leha* - 10-12 gm twice daily with warm milk in empty stomach.
- Daily use of Milk with Ghee (cup of milk with a teaspoon of ghee).

Rasayana for immune-compromised subjects

- *Samshamani Vati* 500 mg tablet, 2 tablet BD after food
- *Agastya Haritaki Rasayana* 10-12 gm BD after food.
- *Chitraka Haritaki Rasayana* 10-12 gm BD after food.
- *Chayavanaprashavaleha* 10-12 gm BD after food.

- *Bramha Rasayana* 10-12 gm BD after food.
- *Swarnamalinivasanta rasa* 125 mg BD after food with water.
- *Guduchi Rasayana* 500 mg BD.

References

1. World Health Organisation Meeting, Geneva, Switzerland, 6–7 February 2012. Preconception care to reduce maternal and childhood mortality and morbidity. Preconception care presentation slides.

   Available from:http://www.who.int/maternal_child_adolescent/ documents/ concensus_preconception_care/en/.
2. Sindhu, RP, Sivaramakrishnapillai, S. Preconception care in Ayurveda. J Indian Sys Medicine 2019; 7: 90-2.
3. Acharya, Y.T. Charaka Samhita of Agnivesha with 'Ayurveda-Dipika' commentary by Chakrapanidatta, Repr. ed. Varanasi. Chaukhamba Surbharati Prakashan. 2000. Sharirasthana, chapter 8, verse 5.
4. Acharya, J.T. and Acharya, N.R. Sushruta Samhita of Sushruta with 'Nibandhasangraha' commentary by Dalhana. Repr. ed. Varanasi. Chaukhamba Surbharati Prakashan. 2003. Sharirasthana, chapter 2, verse 25.
5. Sharma, S. P. Ashtanga Samgraha of VriddhaVagbhata with 'Shashilekha' commentary by Indu. 1st ed. Varanasi. Chowkhamba Sanskrit Series Office. 2006. Sharirasthana, chapter 1, verse 44-45.
6. Acharya, J.T. and Acharya, N.R. Sushruta Samhita of Sushruta with 'Nibandhasangraha' commentary by Dalhana. Repr. ed. Varanasi. Chaukhamba Surbharati Prakashan. 2003. Sharirasthana, chapter 2, verse 33.
7. Roy, A and R. Anjali, Garbhini Ahara, diet during pregnancy, Mahi Publication, Edition first 2020.
8. World Health Organisation (WHO), 2020. Clinical management of COVID-19: interim guidance. 27th May, 2020.
9. Ministry of AYUSH. Government of India. Advisory from Ministry of AYUSH for meeting the challenge arising out of spread of coronavirus (COVID-19) in India. D.O. No. S. 16030/18/2019 – NAM. 6th March. 2020. https://www.ayush.gov.in/docs/125.pdf. (28th May, 2020).
10. Ministry of AYUSH. Government of India. Notification for undertaking research on COVID-19 through Ayurveda, Unani, Siddha and Homoeopathy systems. F.No.L.11011/8/2020/AS. 21st April. 2020. https://www.ayush.gov.in/docs/127.pdf (28th May, 2020).
11. Ministry of AYUSH, Government of India. 'Ayush health promotion product' for commercial manufacturing by Ayurveda, Siddha and Unani drug manufacturers. 24th April 2020. F.No. Z 25023/09/2018-2020-DCC (AYUSH). http://www.ccras.nic.in/sites/default/files/Notices/25042020_Letter_to_States_UTs_for_Ayush_Kwath.pdf (28th May, 2020).
12. Guidelines for Ayurveda Practitioners for COVID 19, GoI, Ministry of AYUSH. Available https://www.ayush.gov.in/docs/ayurveda.pdf (24.10.2020)

4

Food Security Management Strategies: A Perspective from COVID-19 Era

Savitesh Kushwaha, Dr Poonam Khanna, and Dr Rachana Srivastava

Food security is a volatile concept which was redefined and restructured by various organisations since past. The recent and most acceptable definition provided by FAO (Food and Agricultural Organisation) which states that *"food security can be acclaimed when people at all times, have physical and economic access to sufficient, safe and nutritious food that suffice the dietary need of food for sustaining an active and healthy lifestyle"*.The strategic framework for food security works on four pillars – availability, access, utilisation, and stability. Including India, many under-developed and developing countries are currently facing the challenges of food security.[1]

Food Security Status of India

India is self-sufficient to meet the daily dietary and nutritional requirements of the people. After independence, enormous effort has been made to improvise the agricultural system and after the advent of "Green Revolution," India has become self-sufficient in food production. India has enough storage for staples and enough food to procure the nutritional deficiencies, but still struggling to meet the demand and shares a quarter of global hunger burden. In the past 20 years, food production in India has increased from 198 million tonnes to 269 million tonnes with a majority portion consists of wheat and rice. The per capita net availability of food grains and pulses also increases in last decade but still the daily food consumption in both rural and urban areas is lower (1,811 kcal/day and 1,745 kcal/day respectively) than the Indian Council of Medical Research guidelines (2155 kcal/day and 2,090 kcal/day respectively).[1] The huge population burden and lacking strategies to meet the demand of the population is making our way towards several metabolic disorders. The GOI (Government of India) has made several policies and programmes to provide a sufficient amount of dietary components to the Indian population. The PDS (Public Distribution System),which have been observed to reduce the dietary insufficiency through procurement of food grains from the farmers and distributing them at affordable prices to vulnerable sections of the society. The GOI also re-distributes the sufficient amount of food procured through the FCI (Food Corporation of India) to other public welfare schemes like MDM (Mid-Day Meal) scheme for the schools, women and child-related programme, SC/ST hostel etc. The TPDS (Targeted Public Distribution System) of 1997 which is an evolved form of PDS has ensured the delivery of food grains to the poor people[2]. To liquidate the surplus stocks available with the centre and improve the food security the TPDS distribution under AAY increased the limit of 25 kgs per family, per month to 35 kgs per family, per month by the year 2002. The TPDS is an important step in improving the food security in India but also lacked on aspects like leakage, inefficient targeting,biasness, and improper supply chain management. The problems of malnutrition and hunger were continuously pressurising the government to declare a more robust solution to provide food security for all. In wake of this call, the NFSA (National Food Security Act) or *Rashtriya Khadya Suraksha Adhiniyam* was passed by Indian Parliament on 12th September 2013, to make food a legal right so that people can live their life with dignity.[2] It subjected to cover 75% rural and 50% urban population of the country. Currently, the eligible households under Antyodaya Yojana (AAY) Scheme the poorest of the poor are entitled to 5 kgs of food grain per person, per month at the subsidised amount of INR 3 per kg of rice, 2 per kg for wheat and 1 per kg for coarse grains. It is also entitlement for existing food security schemes of India like MDM, ICDS (Integrated Child Development Scheme) and PDS.[3]

To achieve the Sustainable Development Goal 2 by 2030, a timely comprehensive survey is an essential aspect to measure the status of food and nutrition security of the nation. Several national surveys like NFHS-4, NSS, Census and global indexes like GHI (Global Hunger Index) GFSI (Global Food Security Index), Zero Hunger Challenge, Comprehensive Food Security and Vulnerability Analysis (CFSVA) has provided us with the status of food security in India.[1] According to the reports of 2020, India was ranked 94th in GHI and 66th in GFSI.[4,5] In the year 2018-19, FNSA (Food Nutrition Security Analysis) was conducted 2018-2019 to identify the key determinants of food and nutrition security and their multifaceted aspects. This secondary data analysis approach included the several outcomes and indicators influencing food and nutrition security. It included 9 dimensions and 45 variables to assess the status of food and nutrition security in India. 91 million tonnes increased improvement in food grain was reported by FNSA between the year 1996-99 to 2015-2018. The production of cereals wasestimated to be greater than the required and production of pulses has crossed requirement estimate in the year 2016-17.[1] Inspite of sufficient production there are several other factors which are affecting the food and nutrition security in Indiawhich are depicted in the Figure – 1 below.

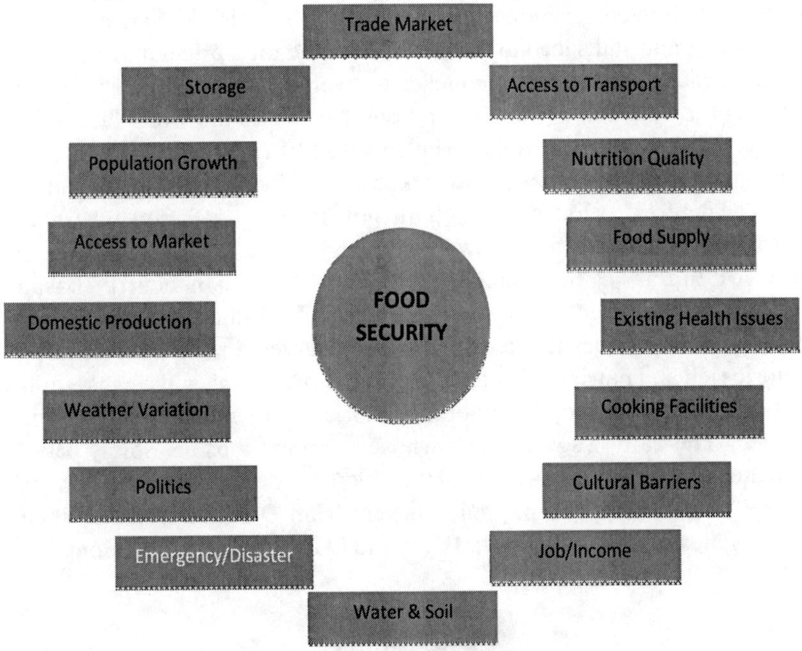

Fig. 1: Factors affecting the food security in India.

Impact of COVID-19 on food security

The World Health Organisation has estimated that the number of people went hungry by the end of 2020 was ~130 million more than the previous year estimate.[6] The pandemic of COVID-19 has nearly limited the Indian food production and supply chain for a certain period. The rigorous lockdown[7] and limited accessibility to food products have affected nearly millions of people across the country. This unplanned emergency has projected already undernourished Indian population to acute hunger situations. The projected Indian economy fall of 9.6% and the unemployment rate of 23.52% was triggered by COVID-19.[8,9] The government has announced the economic package of nearly 10% of GDP but the actual expenditure will be far below than the stated amount.[10]

The limited production, supply, and availability of food dueto COVID-19 have imparted negative effect on all four dimensions of Indian food security (Figure - 2). The COVID-19 outbreak occurs in India during the spring harvesting season called *"Rabi"* which halted the production and sale of the agricultural products like wheat and barley. The lack of availability of farm labours due to returning of migrant labourers to their homes has affected the agricultural production. The closure of restaurants, food places and stalls lead to the downfall in the food prices and wastage. Then a sudden spike in demand leads to overpricing and food shortage.[9] Linking the outbreak to chicken and poultry causes the worst fall in the poultry market in recent times. The shortage of raw materials and high demand for meals at homes due to lockdown was evident among the Indian cities. The fresh food supply chain got severely affected by travel restrictions.[11] The death trolls were also higher due to hunger in several parts of India.[12,13] Increased prevalence of food insecurity hasan unprecedented impact on women and girls.[14] High dietary diversity and fluctuation in calories intake can also be observed among poor peoples. Calorie rich and nutrient-rich food, and other than staples like eggs, fruits and vegetables werecostlier than the calories from staples like rice and maize.[15] The daily wage workers whose consumptions are solely based on per day earning must have faced the severe burden of food procurement for self and family. The migrant workers from Delhi returning to their native states like Uttar Pradesh, Bihar and Odisha have waited alongside

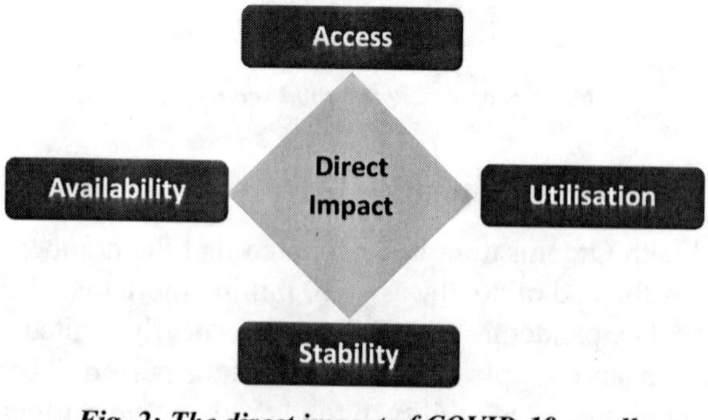

Fig. 2: The direct impact of COVID-19 on all four dimensions of Food Security.

the roads and streets to receive free meals.[16] Several NGOs, independent bodies and institutions were involved in distributing the free meals to the migrant workers and poor peoples who were not able to afford the food during COVID-19 crisis.[17] Disaster relief camps were also setup to help migrants to have access to food and shelter.[18]

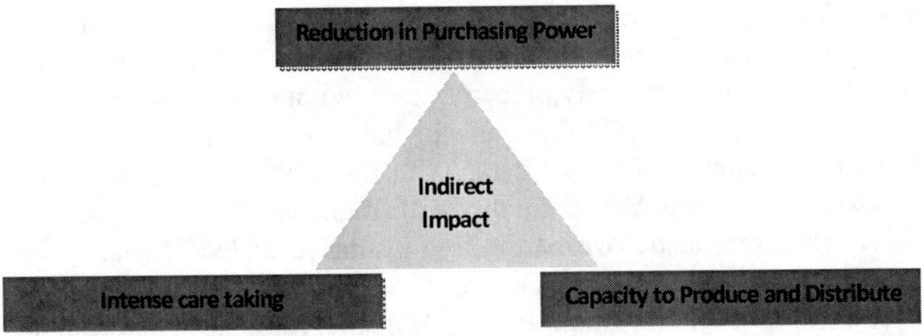

Fig. 3: The indirect impact of COVID-19 on areas related to Food Security.

India's unemployment rate rises to 23.53% amid lockdown during COVID-19 which makes it difficult to buy foods and grains. This increases hunger and reduces purchasing power.[9] The roadways were blocked, and trains and flights were cancelled during the lockdown. After the migrations of millions of daily wage workers and the already produced foods were wasted because of lack of proper storage facilities and lack of affordable transportation for selling and distribution of food products. In turn, decreasing demand due to a decrease in buying power have impacted farmers' and producers' capacity and willingness to invest and implement appropriate technology and also further reduced the production and availability of food. Long-term changes can result in changes in short-term tastes for processed food due to expectations of food safety or comfort, with consequences on food systems, food producers' livelihoods and dietary goods. Overall, a vital juncture in Indian history is the COVID-19 pandemic. For Indian leaders, the evidence-based paths from the rest of the world were helpful for preparedness and taking right steps at the right time to combat the pandemic. Remarkable strategies to secure the livelihoods of millions have been adopted by the bold and determined leadership of both the central and state governments.

Food Security Management Strategies during COVID-19

India is a densely populated country which makes the health management challenging during pandemic situations. Densely populated cities and improper sanitisation require immediate action in response to the spread of the virus. The government officials have taken several measures to curb hunger during COVID-19 pandemic. After the 21 days of the lockdown, the finance minister of India has announced free distribution of extra 5 kg of food grains and 1 kg of pulses per household under Prime Minister Garib Kalyan Ann Yojana for 3 months to beneficiaries covered in NFSA scheme.[19] During the lockdown time, the Food Corporation of India (FCI) ensures uninterrupted supplies of wheat and rice throughout the nation. FCI is completely prepared to meet not only the requirement of food grains under the NFSA beneficiary but also any additional demand, including the supply of 5 Kg / Person to 81.35 Crore individuals under PM Garib Kalyan Ann Yojana for the next 3 months.[20] This relief package of 1.7 lakh crore also covered the free insurance of INR 50 lakhs for frontline healthcare workers.This relief was immediately adopted by several states like Tamil Nadu, Punjab, Haryana, Karnataka, and Andhra Pradesh to deal with the hunger.[18] The INR 1.7 lakh crore tag on the proposed relief package seems impressive, but for FY 2020-21 it is just 5.6 percent of the Union government's projected budget outlay and just 0.8 percent of GDP.[21] Moving a step ahead the government of Kerala announced the distribution of food kits to 87 lakh families till 1st week of April. The chief minister distress relief fund was utilised, and government employees were requested to donate for the relief fund. Each distribution kit costs INR 1000 and was initially distributed among beneficiaries of Antyodaya category. ICAR (Indian Council of Agricultural Research) on 31st March 2020 has issued an advisory to farmers for harvesting *"Rabi"* crops which also included the postharvest storage and marketing of farm-produced.[22] The home delivery system was adopted and telecommunication method was used to contact the beneficiaries.[23] Community kitchen setup was seen among several places like Mumbai,[24] Chandigarh,[25] Kerala,[26] Delhi[27] etc. The local bodies (NGOs) were voluntarily involved in food preparation and distribution whereas the district administration was monitoring the activity. The community kitchen setup was funded by local bodies or state-based industries. The PSUs like Coal India, Adani Foundation, ONGC, BHEL, GAIL, HPLC, CSR, Power Grid, BPCL etc. have donated to PM CARES fund to fight against COVID-19. Other than the food items PSUs were also actively providing LPG cylinders, electricity, petrol, diesel, mask, sanitisers, and other necessary items for running the community kitchens at various places in India.[28] The businessman, celebrities, and individual citizens have also donated to PM CARES funds to curb against COVID-19.[29]

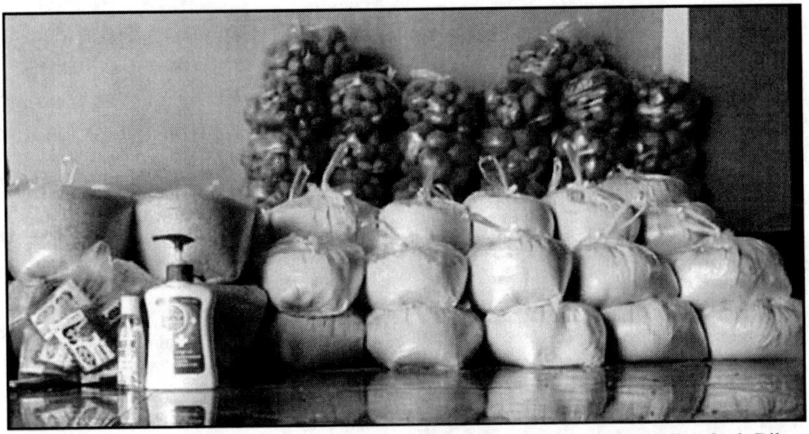

Photo Credits – Ek Roti Team, Jehanabad, Bihar.

Fig. 4: Stocked food and sanitizers for distribution among poor and migrants.

The unsung and unrecognised Anganwadi, ANM (Auxiliary Nurse Midwives) and ASHA (Accredited Social Health Activist) workers during COVID-19 have also shown impeccable determination in maintaining community health. The online training was provided to the Anganwadi workers by the Ministry of Women and Child Development.[30] They continued their duties for new-born babies and pregnant mothers during the pandemic and informed about the necessary preventive measures at the community level. Anganwadi workers were also efficiently educating community people and delivered the *rations* at the doorsteps.[31] However, the difficulties were also faced by people due to the lack of functioning in several places. The closure of Anganwadi centres and schools have limited the dietary intake of several children across the nation.[32] The unpreparedness of pandemic has restricted at least one meal of children who were depended on Anganwadi and MDM. In addition, with mobile COVID-19 testing lab, the DFRL (Defence Food Research Laboratory) have produced nearly 1.5 tonnes of ready to eat foods for healthcare providers in Kochi and Mysuru.[33,34]

Besides these measures, the technologically driven support was also evident in Bengaluru, Karnataka where mobile application *"Homeline"* was launched by the chief minister to deliver groceries and vegetables.[35] Data and information infrastructure technology organisations, such as Impactree, CI Metrices and EDUCO, have joined forces to trace stranded migrant workers in Mumbai. This information is submitted by these organisations to NGOs delivering food in the neighbourhoods where these workers are based. Private sectors companies (Tata group, PepsiCo, and food delivery company like Zomato, The Lalit Hotel group, Nestle India) and NGOs have donated and sponsored meals in government canteens to feed the poor people.[17] NGOs like GOONJ, SEEDS, YUVA, Zomato feeding India, Sharnarthi Sewa, RAHI etc. have provided foods and essentials to millions of labourers and workers.

Table 1: List of Direct Benefit Transfers announced to reduce the burden of COVID-19 and improve food security

Sl. No.	*Direct Benefits to reduce the burden of COVID-19*
1.	Currently, farmers earn INR 6,000/- a year in three equal instalments through the PM-KISAN scheme. For the fiscal year beginning in April 2020, the government will now deliver the first instalment in advance.
2.	MNREGA workers: the rise in salaries from INR 182/- to INR 202/. 50 million families would benefit from such an increase.
3.	For the next three months, 200 million Jan Dhan women account holders will be given an ex-gratia sum of INR 500 per month to run the affairs of their household.
4.	To provide relief to farmers affected by the lockout, the Centre would transfer the first instalment of INR 2,000 to each of the 8.69 crore beneficiaries under the PM-KISAN scheme in the first week of April.
5.	One-time ex-gratia amount of INR 1,000 in two instalments for the next 3 months, 30 million senior citizens, widows, disabled.
6.	Women can receive free LPG cylinders for 3 months in 83 million families below the poverty line protected under the Ujwala system.
7.	The government is doubling collateral-free loans to INR 200,000 for 630,000 self-help groups (SHGs), which assist 70 million households.
8.	State governments have been directed to use the welfare fund for building and construction workers. The District Mineral Fund, worth about INR 310 billion, will be used to help those who are facing economic disruption because of the lockdown.
9.	The government will pay thc Workers' Provident Fund (EPF) contribution, both employer and employee, every month for the next three months. Put together (employee and employer's EPF), that would be 24%.
10.	INR 31,000 crore under the Building and Other Construction Workers' Welfare Cess (BOCW) Act to minimize the effect of the COVID-19 pandemic on 3.5 crore registered workers in their respective state construction worker welfare funds.
11.	INR 15,000 crores New Infrastructure Fund was announced to help COVID-19 affected poultry farms, boost dairy production, and generate jobs.

The Pandemic Lessons

It is beneficial that agricultural and farming activities were not ceased during the pandemic. This help to maintain food security upto a large extent. Losses were faced at several places, but local food agencies helped in the easy flow of food supply and distribution chain which is a commendable task. Although the disruption in transportation services during the lockdown hampered the food security and Indian economy.

The public health policymakers and economists lagged in predicting the exact impact on the health system.In order to prevent the spread of COVID-19, the nation plunges into hunger and malnutrition.

The COVID-19 pandemic has taught several missing aspects of law-making and policy formulation. The ground level monitoring of situation was lacking, the food sector needs wavier and relaxation, coordination between centre and the state government was lacking. The announcement of relief packages has still many questions related to its justification, transfer, and distribution. The cash transfer required detailed information of the recipient which was not possible to obtain in a country where only 2.5% of people pays income tax. The government should build human capacity and infrastructure for job creation in home states. Migration in the search of jobs has claimed many lives in this pandemic. The workers and poor have not even had sufficient earnings to utilise the saving during emergencies. The National Rural Employment Guarantee Act seems to fail in this lockdown. The budget allocation was not sufficient even to meet the daily requirements of workers. One nation and One Ration card should be preferred to facilitate the migration and availability of food for beneficiaries across the nation. Funded by the National Dairy Development Board (NDDB), the Amul model has shown that even during the pandemic crisis, it is possible to protect the livelihoods of small farmers, in this case, milk producers, by concerted action ensuring procurement, storage, transportation, added value and marketing. ICT needs to be strengthened to connect every corner of the country for proper procurement and dispatch of food products.The government require to fasten the policy measures to achieve success in the long term.The future needs to be planned precisely through equally balancing every pillar of food security.

References

1. King, CG. Food and nutrition. Chemical and Engineering News. 1955; 33(1): 29–31.
2. Tanksale, A and Jha, JK. Implementing national food security act in India: Issues and challenges. British Food Journal. 2015; 117(4): 1315–35.
3. Pillay, DPK, Kumar, TKM. Food security in India: Evolution, efforts and problems. Strategic Analysis [Internet]. 2018; 42(6): 595–611. Available from: https://doi.org/10.1080/09700161.2018.1560916
4. Global Food Security Index (GFSI) [Internet]. [cited 2020 Oct 31]. Available from: https://foodsecurityindex.eiu.com/Index

5. India - Global Hunger Index (GHI) - peer-reviewed annual publication designed to comprehensively measure and track hunger at the global, regional, and country levels [Internet]. [cited 2020 Oct 31]. Available from: https://www.globalhungerindex.org/india.html
6. As more go hungry and malnutrition persists, achieving Zero Hunger by 2030 in doubt, UN report warns [Internet]. [cited 2020 Oct 30]. Available from: https://www.who.int/news/item/13-07-2020-as-more-go-hungry-and-malnutrition-persists-achieving-zero-hunger-by-2030-in-doubt-un-report-warns
7. India Lockdown news: India to be under complete lockdown for 21 days starting midnight: Narendra Modi [Internet]. [cited 2020 Oct 30]. Available from: https://economictimes.indiatimes.com/news/politics-and-nation/india-will-be-under-complete-lockdown-starting-midnight-narendra-modi/articleshow/74796908.cms
8. GDP India | Why projected 9.5% fall in GDP makes this the worst recession in Indian history – and what it means | Business News [Internet]. [cited 2020 Oct 30]. Available from: https://www.timesnownews.com/business-economy/economy/article/why-projected-9-5-fall-in-gdp-makes-this-the-worst-recession-in-indian-history-and-what-it-means/665991
9. Organização das NaçõesUnidas (ONU). Impact of COVID-19 on food security and nutrition (FSN). United Nations [Internet]. 2020;(March):1–8. Available from: http://www.ceigram.upm.es/wp-content/uploads/2020/03/HLPE.-Impact-of-COVID-19-on-FSN-2020-03-24.pdf
10. Narendra Modi: PM Narendra Modi announces Rs 20 lakh crore economic package, BFSI News, ET BFSI [Internet]. [cited 2020 Oct 31]. Available from: https://bfsi.economictimes.indiatimes.com/news/industry/pm-narendra-modi-announces-rs-20-lac-crore-economic-package/75699302
11. Covid-19 puts India's food supply chain to a stress-test - The Hindu Business Line [Internet]. [cited 2020 Oct 30]. Available from: https://www.thehindubusinessline.com/economy/agri-business/covid-19-puts-indias-food-supply-chain-to-a-stress-test/article31173973.ece
12. Coronavirus-linked hunger tied to 10,000 child deaths each month - World News [Internet]. [cited 2020 Oct 30]. Available from: https://www.indiatoday.in/world/story/coronavirus-linked-hunger-tied-to-10-000-child-deaths-each-month-1705144-2020-07-28
13. More than 300 Indians have died of the coronavirus, and nearly 200 of the lockdown [Internet]. [cited 2020 Oct 30]. Available from: https://theprint.in/opinion/more-than-300-indians-have-died-of-the-coronavirus-and-nearly-200-of-the-lockdown/400714/
14. COVID-19 will worsen the already abysmal state of nutrition among women - Nutrition International [Internet]. [cited 2020 Oct 30]. Available from: https://www.nutritionintl.org/2020/06/covid-19-will-worsen-the-already-abysmal-state-of-nutrition-among-women/
15. Headey, DD, Alderman, HH. The Relative Caloric Prices of Healthy and Unhealthy Foods Differ Systematically across Income Levels and Continents. Journal of Nutrition [Internet]. 2019 Nov 1 [cited 2020 Oct 30];149(11):2020–33. Available from: https://doi.org/10.1093/jn/nxz158.

16. The Coronavirus Lockdown Has Been a War on India's Informal Labour [Internet]. [cited 2020 Oct 30]. Available from: https://thewire.in/labour/coronavirus-lockdown-informal-labour
17. List of NGOs providing relief during Covid-19 [Internet]. [cited 2020 Oct 30]. Available from: https://www.investindia.gov.in/bip/resources/list-ngos-providing-relief-during-covid-19
18. Local food systems and COVID-19; A glimpse on India's responses | Food for the cities programme | Food and Agriculture Organization of the United Nations [Internet]. [cited 2020 Oct 30]. Available from: http://www.fao.org/in-action/food-for-cities-programme/news/detail/en/c/1272232/
19. Govt to give extra 5 kg grains, 1 kg pulses for free under PDS for next 3 months: FM Nirmala Sitharaman - The Economic Times [Internet]. [cited 2020 Oct 31]. Available from: https://economictimes.indiatimes.com/news/economy/policy/govt-to-provide-5-kg-grains-1-kg-pulses-for-free-over-next-3-months-fm/articleshow/74827003.cms?from=mdr
20. FCI ensures uninterrupted food grain supplies across the country during the lockdown due to COVID-19 outbreak [Internet]. [cited 2020 Oct 31]. Available from: https://pib.nic.in/PressReleseDetail.aspx?PRID=1610732
21. Nine Concerns About the Centre's 1.7 Lakh Crore Package [Internet]. [cited 2020 Oct 31]. Available from: https://thewire.in/government/covid-19-india-government-package
22. Welfare F, Council TI. In wake of COVID-19 spread, ICAR issues Advisory to farmers for Rabi crops. 2020.
23. Kerala starts free food grain supply; seeks a month's salary from government employees - Frontline [Internet]. [cited 2020 Oct 31]. Available from: https://frontline.thehindu.com/dispatches/article31229663.ece
24. Covid-19 lockdown: In India, community kitchens spring across cities to feed stranded migrants [Internet]. [cited 2020 Oct 31]. Available from: https://scroll.in/article/958366/covid-19-in-india-community-kitchens-spring-up-across-cities-to-feed-stranded-migrants
25. Community kitchen to serve the needy/: The Tribune India [Internet]. [cited 2020 Oct 31]. Available from: https://www.tribuneindia.com/news/chandigarh/community-kitchen-to-serve-the-needy-65781
26. Fighting COVID-19: Community Kitchens In Thiruvananthapuram Deliver Food To 67,000 Migrants And Poor Amid Lockdown [Internet]. [cited 2020 Oct 31]. Available from: https://special.ndtv.com/coronavirus-61/news-detail/fighting-covid-19-community-kitchens-in-thiruvananthapuram-deliver-food-to-67-000-migrants-and-poor-2215652/7
27. From Community Kitchen to PPE: How Indians Showed Solidarity with Covid-19 Affected [Internet]. [cited 2020 Oct 31]. Available from: https://www.news18.com/news/buzz/from-community-kitchen-to-ppe-how-indians-showed-solidarity-with-covid-19-affected-2578797.html
28. Maharatna PSUs have contributed a hefty Rs 1,577 cr via CSR to PM CARES [Internet]. [cited 2020 Oct 31]. Available from: https://psuwatch.com/maharatna-psus-have-contributed-a-hefty-rs-1577-cr-via-csr-to-pm-cares

29. PM CARES gets Rs 6,500 crore donation in a week, 3 times more than what PMNRF got in 2 yrs [Internet]. [cited 2020 Oct 31]. Available from: https://theprint.in/india/pm-cares-gets-rs-6500-crore-donation-in-a-week-3-times-more-than-what-pmnrf-got-in-2-yrs/395172/
30. Anganwadi workers get online sessions on COVID-19 steps - The Hindu [Internet]. [cited 2020 Oct 31]. Available from: https://www.thehindu.com/news/national/anganwadi-workers-get-online-sessions-on-covid-19-steps/article31264237.ece
31. Unsung, Unrecognised, Anganwadi Workers Protect The Most Vulnerable | Outlook Poshan [Internet]. [cited 2020 Oct 31]. Available from: https://poshan.outlookindia.com/story/poshan-news-unsung-unrecognised-they-protect-the-most-vulnerable/355312
32. India Coronavirus Dispatch: Anganwadis shut down; schools prepare to reopen | Business Standard News [Internet]. [cited 2020 Oct 31]. Available from: https://www.business-standard.com/article/current-affairs/india-coronavirus-dispatch-anganwadis-shut-down-schools-prepare-to-reopen-120091101031_1.html
33. From Gaganyaan to COVID-19: DFRL provides quick meals for healthcare workers - The Week [Internet]. [cited 2020 Oct 31]. Available from: https://www.theweek.in/news/india/2020/04/10/from-gaganyaan-to-covid-19-dfrl-provides-quick-meals-for-healthcare-workers.html
34. DFRL develops mobile COVID-19 testing lab - The Hindu [Internet]. [cited 2020 Oct 31]. Available from: https://www.thehindu.com/news/national/karnataka/dfrl-develops-mobile-covid-19-testing-lab/article31556581.ece
35. Karnataka launches app for home delivery of essentials in Bengaluru [Internet]. [cited 2020 Oct 31]. Available from: https://www.livemint.com/news/india/karnataka-launches-app-for-home-delivery-of-essentials-in-bengaluru-11587483300833.html

5

Ayurveda in Understanding and Managing Covid-19: During and post-Covid era

Dr Binay Sen

It is almost a year, the entire world has been fighting against an infectious disease known as the novel coronavirus disease 2019 (Covid-19), caused by an RNA virus SARS-CoV-2 (Severe Acute Respiratory Syndrome coronavirus-2). The World Health Organization (WHO) has declared it as a pandemic in March 2020. As on 25th October 2020, WHO has reported over 42 million cases and 1.1 million deaths worldwide. In India, as on 29th October 2020, the total confirmed cases figured to 80,40,203 with 1,20,527 deaths.

Presently, the conventional management of Covid-19 relies on prophylaxis and symptomatic intervention with life supporting care in critically ill patients. Various existing drugs are being repurposed for the clinical use, new targets are being identified every day, and numerous drugs are also undergoing clinical trials along with vaccines. The frequent alterations in the antigenic structures (viral strain) of respiratory RNA virus (as in COVID-19) posed further difficulties in its addressal. Even though vaccines against SARS-CoV-2 have come, prevention from getting infected by the virus and enhancing the host immunity to minimise the morbidity and mortality remain as the main aim of the health fraternity. It is essential to find a long-term solution to live in COVID era by adopting a holistic approach to prevent or cure of physical, psychological, social and spiritual suffering. Ayurveda takes care of total health of an individual by advocating different regimens as described under *dinacharya* (daily regimen), *ritucharya* (seasonal regimen), *sadvritta* (code of conduct), *achara rasayana* (behavioural rejuvenating therapy) for prevention and disease specific customised approach for managing the disease.

The Ministry of AYUSH has introduced measures to manage the outbreak of Covid-19 through different preventive and prophylactic measures like improving the immunity and symptomatic intervention through simple remedies made of common medicinal plants (used in symptoms like COVID-19).

Ayurveda in understanding Covid-19

To understand the role of Ayurvedic management in pandemic like Covid-19, it is essential to understand the concept of newly emerging disease, origin of epidemic/pandemic and mode of transmission of communicable diseases. The vitiated *dosha* (body humour) causes various disorders according to variation in *vikara-prakriti* (the natural course of disease), *samutthana* (etiological component) and *adhishthana* (location/ the site of pathological involvement). Hence every disease could not be assigned with name and management of newly emerging disease is based on the above factors [*Charaka Samhita. Sutrasthana.* chapter 18. verse 42-45].

An epidemic occurring over a very wide geographical area, crossing the international boundaries, affecting a large number of population, significantly increasing morbidity and mortality, disrupting socio-economic and political harmony, is known as pandemic. It is stated that epidemic disorders caused due to polluted *vayu* (air), *ap* (water), *desha* (habitat) and *kala* (season), which has a direct causal relationship with *pragyaparadha* (intellectual errors) as referred under *janapadodhvansa* (epidemics) [*Charaka Samhita. Vimanasthana.* Chapter. 3]. *Pragya* means 'intelligence'and *aparadha* means 'misconduct' or 'offence'. It is the root of all diseases as described in *Ayurveda.* It is defined as the errors in one's *dhee* (intellect), *dhriti* (restraint) and *smriti* (memory) lead to improper activities of body (physical), mind (mental) and speech (verbal) leading to vitiation of all *doshas* resulting in manifestation of somatic or psycho-somatic diseases. In *Sushruta Samhita*, the modes of human-to-human transmission of communicable diseases are mentioned as physical contact, exhalation, eating together in same plate, sharing bed, using clothes, garlands, and paste. Improper *ahara* (diet) and wrong *vihara* (behaviour) negatively influence healthy status of the body, mind, and sense organs. These concepts are very much relevant with the origin, disease spread, mode of transmission, disease severity and post-Covid impact. These all give a strong fundamental approach to understand epidemic/pandemic in Ayurveda and design management protocol accordingly.

Symptoms

According to the Centers for Disease Control and Prevention (CDC), people with COVID-19 have had a wide range of symptoms ranging from mild symptoms to severe illness. Symptoms may appear within 2-14 days after exposure to the virus. People with these symptoms may have COVID-19:

- Fever or chills
- Cough
- Shortness of breath or difficulty breathing
- Fatigue
- Muscle or body aches
- Headache
- New loss of taste or smell
- Sore throat
- Congestion or runny nose
- Nausea or vomiting
- Diarrhea.

In Ayurveda, the newly emerging Covid-19 can be categorised under *agantujavyadhi* (exogenous disease) by origin, caused by *bhoota* (micro-organisms), and on due course transforming to *nija* (endogenous) disease leading to disequilibrium of *kapha*, *vata* and *pittadosha*s with psycho-somatic involvement. The analysis of clinical manifestation and ongoing disease progression, it is well considered as *vata-kaphapradhanatridoshajavyadhi* that mainly involves *pranavaha* (cardio-pulmonary system), *rasavaha* (cardio-vascular system) and *raktavaha* (vascular and reticuloendothelial system) *srotas* and the disease located to the respiratory system. In severe condition, it diminishes the *agni* and *ojas* involving multiple *srotas* system (multi-organ failure) leading to death.

Ayurveda in managing Covid-19

Ayurveda is a science of life and arts of living. It is so called Ayurveda as it imparts knowledge about the substances (used in forms of diet and drugs) along with their properties and actions, aiming at to prevent the disease occurrence and maintain the health of healthy individual through its holistic approach of *ahara* (dietetic), *vihara* (lifestyle) and *aushadha* (pharmacotherapy) intervention. This three-fold intervention is also applicable in Covid-19 considering the *ayushya* (conducive) and *anayushya* (unconducive) to the patient.

Nidanaparivarjana (avoiding etiological components)

It is the foremost non-pharmacological intervention for any ailment (*Sushruta Samhita. Uttaratantra.* Chapter 1. verse 25) and very specific to infectious disease. The best way to avoid those habits or practices through which the transmission of virus takes place or which may lead to respiratory tract susceptible for infection. Touching face and nose, spitting in public place, cold/ iced food and drinks, crowded area to be avoided.

Maintaining *agni* (digestive/metabolic fire)

Agni is the digestive and metabolic fire that plays an important role in *jatharagni-paka* (gastrointestinal digestion), *bhootagni* and *dhatwagnipaka* (cellular metabolism). Any metabolic reaction including the digestion, absorption and assimilation of food and drinks are under the control of *agni*. It is well explained that lifespan, strength, health, immunity, vital breath etc depend on normal body-fire and its derangement leads to disease condition, even death. Hence, maintenance of *agni* is important to boost up immunity and reserve the vital breath in Covid-19 patients also. Drugs categorised under *deepana* (that stimulates *agni*) and *pachana* (promotes gastric secretion for digestion) like *Pippali* (*Piper longum*/ Long pepper), *Maricha* (*Piper nigrum*/ Black pepper), *Shunthi* (*Zingiber officinale*/ dried ginger); collectively known as *Trikatu*, *Yavani* (*Trachyspermumammi*/ Ajowan), *Jeeraka* (*Cuminum cyminum*/ Cumin seed), *Hingu* (*Ferula narthex*/ Asafoetida) easily available in Indian kitchen are used for the above purpose.

Ahara (diet and drinks)

Ayurveda believes that all the diseases are primarily due to a faulty digestion. It is advised to have easily digestible foods rich in green seasonal vegetables and fruits. Citrus fruit is considered healthy due to vitamin-C, an antioxidant, essential for immunity and free radical scavenging. Drinking warm water stimulates hunger; it plays an important role in digestion. It is ideal for those suffering from new fever, cough, dyspnoea, coryza and pain in flanks. Some herbs like *Adrak* (fresh ginger), *Tulasi* (*Ocimum sanctum*/Holy basil), *Dalchini* (*Cinnamomum zeylanicum*/ Cinnamon), *Tejpatra* (*Cinnamomum tamala*/ Bay leaf), *Lavanga* (*Syzygiumaromaticum*/ Clove) and *Maricha* which could be used singly or in combination to prepare hot infusion/tea that capable of reducing *kaphadosha* and fight against micro-organism. This is also helpful in sorethroat. Some spices- *Haridra* (*Curcuma longa*/Turmeric), *Hingu, Lasuna* (*Allium sativum*/ Garlic), *Ela* (*Elettaria cardamomum*/ Lesser cardamom), *Javitri* (seed aril of *Myristica fragrans*/ Mace), Cumin seed, Coriander seed are commonly used in Indian cuisine. These Ayurvedic medicinal plants are having multiple therapeutic indices with antioxidant, antihyperlipidaemic, antidiabetic, fibrinolytic, antiviral, stimulant, digestive and carminative action. Avoiding intake of high calorie fatty, spicy, fast and junk foods is equally important.

Studies reported that alkaline environment within the normal range of blood pH (7.35 to 7.45) positively influences the inflammatory, immune and antiviral responses of the body. It means that in an alkaline environment, chemotaxis, phagocytosis and bactericidal capacity of polymorphonuclear leukocytes might be enhanced, immune function may work better and the virus might be weakened or replication hampered. The alkalinity of the blood pH towards its normal upper limit (7.45) can be achieved through increasing alkaline dietary sources or alkaline drinks (predominantly fruits and vegetables) and reducing acidic dietary sources (meat, fish, eggs, dairy products, grains and grain products, soft drinks etc.) [Mousa HA, 2017].

Vihara (lifestyle modifications)

As the virus spreads most commonly from an infected person to others through respiratory droplets produced when an infected person coughs or sneezes, close personal contact, or touching an object or surface contaminated with the virus and then touching mouth or nose before washing hands. Thus, the personal and social hygiene play an important role in preventing disease spread. The need for social distancing is essential and hence the various world leaders implemented stringent lockdowns in most parts of the world at the initial stage of the pandemic. General precautions like not spitting in public places, use of mask, frequent hand washing with soap and rubbing with alcohol-based sanitizer, avoid touching of face and nose are all about to prevent the spread and contamination of the virus.

Regular exercise, *yogasana*, *pranayama*, meditation stimulate the immune system by increasing blood circulation, stimulating the lymphatic system and decreasing stress hormones. Daytime sleep is to be avoided as it leads to *kapha* accumulation. Exposure to dust, pollen, mites and other allergens to be avoided to keep the respiratory system healthy.

Aushadha (pharmacotherapy/drugs)

The principle of treatment for any newly emerging disease is designed on the basis of nature (epidemic/pandemic), etiology (microorganism) and location (the respiratory system) of the disorder [Charaka Samhita. Sutrasthana, chapter 18, verse 46]. For an epidemic disease, use of *rasayana* drugs [Charaka Samhita. Vimanasthana, chapter 3, verse 14], disinfectants for microorganism [Sushruta Samhita. Sutrasthana, chapter 5, verse 18] and disease-location specific treatment i.e. anti-cough, anti-dyspnoea, anti-pyretic, stimulant and digestive drugs will be effective in this condition. Apart from these, *rasayana* drugs acting on *rasavaha*, *pranavaha* and *raktavahasrotas* like *Guduchi* (*Tinospora cordifolia*/ Giloy; taken in form of hot infusion of fresh stem/ *Samshamanivati*/ *Guduchighanvati*), *Pippali*, *Haritaki* (*Terminalia chebula*/ Chebulic myrobalan), *Amalaki* (*Emblica officinalis*/ Indian gooseberry), *Bhallataka* (*Semecarpus anacardium*/ Marking nut) are used in treating ailments like fever, cough, dysponea, bodyache, indigestion, loss of appetite etc. *Rasayana* drug is claimed to have *ojas* (immunity) enhancing property and hence effective in prophylaxis of many viral diseases including Covid-19. The drugs listed in the advisory by the AYUSH Ministry are common medicinal plants useful in similar symptoms like *Ashwagandha* (*Withaniasomnifera*/ Indian ginseng), *Yashthimadhu* (*Glycyrrhiza glabra*/ Liquorice root), *Tulasi*, *Guduchi*, Ginger and Turmeric. The '*AyushKwath*' (Table 1) consists of *Tulsi*, *Dalchini*, *Shunthi* and *Maricha*, is an immunity boosting measure, adopted during this Covid-19 outbreak. Most of the drugs mentioned above are hot in nature and may cause gastric upset, constipation, eruptions on the skin etc in some individuals. Hence it is recommended to take these medicines under the supervision of Ayurvedic physician. It is better to add *Mulethi* (*yashthimadhu*), *Amalaki*, *Draksha* and *Mishri* while preparing decoction or tea with the above medicines. There is an important seasonal *rasayana* therapy referred in Ayurveda as '*Ritu-Haritaki*', which rejuvenates in different seasons (Table 2).

Table 1: *Ayush Kwatha* ingredients, preparation and modes of administration

Sl. No.	*Ingredients*	*Part taken*	*Quantity*
1.	*Tulsi* (*Ocimum sanctum*)	Leaf	4 parts
2.	*Dalchini* (*Cinnamomum zeylanicum*)	Stem bark	2 parts
3.	*Shunthi* (*Zingiber officinale*)	Rhizome	2 parts
4.	*Krishna Maricha* (*Piper nigrum*)	Fruit	1 part
Method of preparation and use	Take all the standard ingredients in dry form and make coarse powder. Take 3 grams of powder to be consumed like tea or hot drink by dissolving in 150 ml of boiled water, once or twice daily. *Guda* (jaggery) / *Draksha* (resins) and/or Lemon Juice can be added while consuming the formulation.		

Table 2: *Ritu-Haritaki* (*Bhavaprakasha Nighantu. Haritakyadi Varga*. verse no. 34)

Sl. No.	*Season*	*Adjuvant*
1.	*Varsha Ritu* – Monsoon (mid July-mid September)	*Saindhava* (Rock salt)
2.	*Sharad Ritu* – Autumn (mid September-mid November)	*Sharkara* (*Mishri*)
3.	*Hemanta Ritu* – Early Winter (mid November-mid January)	*Shunthi* (Dried ginger powder)
4.	*Shishira Ritu* – Winter (mid January-mid March)	*Pippali* (Long pepper powder)
5.	*Vasanta Ritu* – Spring (mid March-mid May)	*Madhu* (Honey)
6.	*Grishma Ritu* – Summer (mid May-mid July)	*Guda* (Jaggery)
Method of Preparation and use	Take 3 gm of *Haritaki* (without seed) powder and mixed with equal quantity of adjuvant as per season, once or twice daily.	

Pratimarsha-nasya (nasal smearing)

Pratimarsha-nasya (smearing the nostrils with oil) is a type of nasal therapy described in Ayurveda and also traditionally in practice. It is applied through one's finger dipped into oil on to the nasal mucosa every day morning and night without expelling it out. Instilling two drops of sesame oil in each nostril every morning can be used to prevent the new coronavirus. Studies reported that applying sesame oil prevents direct contact and binding of virus onto the surface of nasal mucosa, suppresses the coronavirus replication. Thus, this may prevent transmission to the lower respiratory tract and other human. [Wen, F. *et al.,* 2020; Yan, Bingpeng, *et al.,* 2019]. It is also reported that coconut oil is having antiviral activity against the novel coronavirus [Fabian M. D. and Mary T. N. 2020)]. This nasal medication of oil diminishes *vata* (hyper-responsiveness) and *kapha* (responsible for hyper-secretion), thus maintains naso-pharyngeal healthy muco-ciliary activity.

Kavala (gargling)

It is reported that the Covid-19 virus initially lodges in to the mucosa of upper respiratory tract (mouth, oro-pharynx and naso-pharynx), from where it transmits into the lower respiratory system or other humans through infectious droplets. Hence, nasal smearing and gurgling may be effective to prevent further progression as well as transmission of virus. Turmeric powder with rock salt (both one pinch) added in warm water (100 ml) is commonly advocated for this purpose.

Chewing of *Tamboola/* (*Piper betel/* Betel leaf) leaf with *Jaatiphala* (*Myristica fragrans/* Nutmeg seed), *Lavanga* is also good for maintain oral and upper respiratory hygiene.

Post-Covid management

It comprises both physical and psychological intervention to support the psycho-somatic system for normal functioning.

Use of *Deepana, Pachana, Balya, Brimhana, Rasayana* therapies

After getting cured from any disease, Ayurveda recommends light diets along with proper prescription of *pathya* (do's) and *apathya* (don'ts). It is because the digestive fire remains in subduing stage and body tissues become relatively weak. Hence stimulant and digestive drugs, medicated soups etc given to strengthen the *agni* followed by strength (*balya*) and bulk (*brimhana*) promoting measures (nutritious diets, herbs like *Bala, Ashwagandha, Shatavari* and *Vidarikanda* powder). So that, the body system gets healthy and immune to prevent from remission and relapse of disease further. *Rasayana* drugs also give strength to the body, enrich body cells and systems and provide immunity against diseases.

Stress management and improving socio-psychological health

Any pandemic is a state of emergency and in such diverse situation all individuals are often exposed to potentially traumatic events, that subsequently imbalance the behavioural, emotional, social and somatic reactions. Evidence also suggests that individuals may experience symptoms of psychosis, anxiety, trauma, suicidal tendency, and panic during outbreaks of communicable diseases. Anxiety is a facilitator of decreased immune response to infection and further increases the severity of the disease. Various stressors have culminated to breakdown in normal functioning of the individuals. Unemployment, increased financial strain, uncertainty in academic calendar and the fear of the post-Covid complication all put a person across the limits of his/her psychological well-being. Unless an established mental disorder, most of the psycho-somatic reactions are well managed and controlled through the non-pharmacological interventions.

Stress and anxiety produce acidic pH, which negatively influences many intracellular and extracellular functions of the body, while meditation and exercise leading to alkaline pH of the blood [Mousa HA, 2017]. Therefore, one should avoid the stressors like excessive exposure to media coverage of COVID-19 that creates lot of anxiety and panic. It is better to access information resources of the Health organisations (WHO, CDC, NIH, MoAYUSH, MoHFW) that provide awareness about how to protect oneself and family from getting infected. Try to do some other productive activities like taking up new hobbies. Eat healthy and well-balanced traditional home made meals. Deep breathing exercise, meditation, proper sleep (7-8 hours night sleep with regular sleeping and waking time), listening to calm music, prayers impart soothing effect to the mind. Maintain healthy family and friend relationships. Avoid alcohol, smoking and any abusive drugs. Any persistence disturbance in the mental wellbeing, consult physician or psychiatrist for timely management.

Conclusion

Ayurveda emphasises on preventive and restorative health more strongly than curing any ailments. Proper diets, healthy lifestyle and rejuvenation according to season, place, body constitution are the way to prevent diseases occurrence, and in addition to pharmacotherapy, effective in managing diseases. Common medicinal plants/ products those available in home garden/ kitchen are rich in many pharmacological properties with nutrition values. Rational administration of drugs along with practice of *pathya* and *apathya* in form of *ahara*, *vihara* and *achara* are the keys of Ayurvedic holistic approach towards health and disease, which also applicable in during Covid-19 outbreak and post-Covid era.

References

1. World Health Organization (WHO). Weekly epidemiological update - 27 October 2020.https://www.who.int/publications/m/item/weekly-epidemiological-update—27-october-2020 (Accessed on 28th October 2020).
2. Government of India. IndiaFightsCorona COVID-19 in India. 29th October. 2020. https://www.mygov.in/covid-19.
3. *Charaka Samhita.* Available from: http://niimh.nic.in/ebooks/echarak (Accessed on 25th October 2020).
4. *Sushruta Samhita.* Available from: http://niimh.nic.in/ebooks/esushruta (Accessed on 25th October 2020).
5. Centers for Disease Control and Prevention (CDC). Symptoms of Coronavirus Disease 2019. https://www.cdc.gov/coronavirus/2019-ncov/symptoms-testing/symptoms.html (Accessed on 27th October 2020).
6. Sen Binay. Potentiality and possibility of Medicinal Plants on Ayurvedic Principle in prevention and treatment of COVID-19. 2020;6. 100-107. doi:10.31254/jahm.2020.6216.
7. Sharma, P. V. *DravyagunaVijnana*, Vol. 2. Reprint Edition. Chaukhambha Bharati Academy, Varanasi, 1998.

8. Bhavaprakasa Nighantu. Reprint Edition. Commentary by K.C. Chunekar, Edited by Dr G.S. Pandey, Chaukhambha Bharati Academy, Varanasi, 2004.
9. Binay Sen. COVID-19: A disease targeted drug review of plant origin in Ayurveda. Journal of Vishwa Ayurved Parishad. May-June 2020. Year 17, Vol. 5-6; 51-62.
10. Mousa, HA. Prevention and Treatment of Influenza, Influenza-Like Illness, and Common Cold by Herbal, Complementary, and Natural Therapies. *J Evid Based Complementary Altern Med.* 2017;22(1):166-174. doi:10.1177/2156587216641831. (Accessed on 28th October 2020).
11. Ministry of AYUSH. Government of India. Advisory from Ministry of AYUSH for meeting the challenge arising out of spread of coronavirus (COVID-19) in India. D.O. No. S. 16030/18/2019 – NAM. 6th March. 2020. https://www.ayush.gov.in/docs/125.pdf. (Accessed on 28th October 2020).
12. Ministry of AYUSH. Government of India. Ayurveda's immunity boosting measures for self care during COVID-19 crisis. Available from: https://www.ayush.gov.in/docs/123.pdf.(Accessed on 28th October 2020).
13. Ministry of AYUSH, Government of India. 'Ayush health promotion product' for commercial manufacturing by Ayurveda, Siddha and Unani drug manufacturers. 24th April 2020. F.No. Z 25023/09/2018-2020-DCC (AYUSH). http://www.ccras.nic.in/sites/default/files/Notices/25042020_Letter_to_States_UTs_for_Ayush_Kwath.pdf.(Accessed on 28th October 2020).
14. Ministry of AYUSH. AYUSH Advisory for Corona virus 2020. 29th Jan. 2020 https://pib.gov.in/PressReleasePage.aspx?PRID=1600895(Accessed on 28th October 2020).
15. Wen, F., Jing, Z., Yunfeng, X. A theoretical discussion of the possibility and possible mechanisms of using sesame oil for prevention of 2019-nCoV (Wuhan coronavirus) from the perspective of colloid and interface science, 2020. DOI: 10.13140/RG.2.2.31786.98248. https://www.researchgate.net/publication/339123581(Accessed on 28th October 2020).
16. Yan, Bingpeng, et al. "Characterization of the lipidomic profile of human coronavirus-infected cells: Implications for lipid metabolism remodeling upon coronavirus replication." Viruses. 2019. 11.1; 73.]. (Accessed on 27th October 2020).
17. Fabian, M. D. and Mary, T. N. The potential of coconut oil and its derivatives as effective and safe antiviral agents against the novel coronavirus (nCov-2019). 2020. https://ateneo.edu/ls/sose/sose/news/research/potential-coconut-oil-and-its-derivatives-effective-and-safe-antiviral(Accessed on 28th October 2020).
18. Handbook of Mental Health issues during Covid-19 pandemic. 1st Edition, 2020, published by department of psychiatry, IMS, BHU, Varanasi.

6

Therapeutic Potential of Dietary Phytonutrients against COVID-19

Dr Shachi Singh

Recent attack of Corona virus has severely affected human population, taking life of more than 2 million people around the globe. Lack of effective therapeutic agents prompted the scientists to look for various alternative measures, which can inhibit the spread of the disease or reduce its severity. Compounds present in chemical libraries as well as in natural isolates have been searched against the virus. It had been observed that several phytonutrients present in our daily diet can have the potential to fight against the disease. Many foods when tested against COVID-19 showed promising results. Phytonutrients such as polyphenols, vitamins and minerals like selenium and zinc have shown to provide protection from the virus by either acting as antiviral agents or as immunomodulators. In this chapter, role of some important functional foods and phytonutrients have been discussed which help in combating the disease.

In December 2019, cases of COVID-19 were first reported from the city of Wuhan, China, and since then millions of people around the world have been infected and many have lost their life in the battle against the disease (Pedersen and Ho, 2020). COVID-19 is a viral disease caused by severe acute respiratory syndrome corona virus (SARS-CoV-2) (Islam *et al.,* 2020). The virus belongs to a diverse family of Corona viruses that infect a wide range of avian and mammalian hosts (Brian and Baric, 2005). Some mammalian species such as bats and birds were the natural host of corona viruses, however host range expansion had been observed during its evolutionary history, and as a result, human corona viruses have emerged as zoonotic pathogens (Lu *et al.,* 2020). Severe acute respiratory syndrome corona virus (SARS-CoV), Middle East respiratory syndrome corona virus (MERS-CoV) and the recent one SARS-CoV-2 are some examples of severe pathogenic forms of human coronavirus (Islam *et al.*, 2020; Chafekar and Fielding, 2018).

SARS-CoV-2 mainly infects the respiratory system, but can also progress to various other organs thereby affecting digestive system, circulatory system, nervous system and urogenital system (Huang *et al.*, 2020). Viral infection is transmitted predominately by respiratory droplets generated when people cough, sneeze, talk, or breathe. Virus particles penetrate the host tissues through the mucous membrane of the respiratory tract and begin to replicate. As a result, respiratory tract swells and get inflamed. After that viral particles enter the lungs and then to the bloodstream, from where they spread the infection throughout the body. Once the infection spreads more symptoms begin to show. Most common are fever, dry cough, runny nose, difficulty in breathing, pneumonia and diarrhea. The disease in severe cases may ultimately cause multiple organ failure and can lead to death in some cases (Chen *et al.,* 2020). Older people and those with pre-existing medical conditions such as diabetes, cardiovascular and chronic respiratory problems are much vulnerable than others (Huang *et al.,* 2020; Chen *et al.,* 2020; Lim, 2004).

In the current situation, measures to control infection are crucial for disease management. Several preventive measures have been advised for general public health including, hand and respiratory hygiene, use of masks, self-quarantine etc (WHO, 2020). Scientists around the globe have worked on finding a cure for the disease in the form of a vaccine or antiviral agents. Various natural products have also evolved as a cure and people are looking back towards our traditional medicinal system to combat the adverse effect of the disease (Chojnacka *et al.,* 2020; Islam *et al.,* 2020). Currently various functional foods and neutraceuticals have been validated for their role against the virus. It has been observed that many dietary phytochemicals and micronutrients can help individuals to overcome the infection by either modulating the immune system or generating some antiviral activity against the disease or controlling other health problems arising due to the infection (Sahebnasagh *et al.,* 2020).

About the virus

SARS COV-2 are enveloped, spherical shaped single-stranded, positive-sense RNA viruses of diameter 50–200 nanometres and genome size of 26.4–31.7 kb (Brian and Baric, 2005; Lu *et al.,* 2020). The genome encodes 16 nonstructural proteins, including proteases, RNA- dependent RNA polymerase, RNA helicase, primase, and others, required to synthesize viral mRNAs. The genome encodes four structural proteins, namely the spike protein (S), envelope protein (E), membrane protein (M), and nucleocapsid protein (N). The N protein holds the RNA genome, and the S, E, and M proteins together create the viral envelope (Lu *et al.*, 2020). The club-shaped projections from the viral envelope resembling a crown is made of spike protein. The spike protein, is also responsible for the attachment of the virus to the host cell membrane (Lu *et al.*, 2020). The receptor for both SARS-CoV and SARS-CoV-2 is angiotensin-converting enzyme 2 (ACE2), a cell-surface enzyme (Xu *et al.*, 2020). A higher rate of SARS-CoV-2 infections compared with SARS-CoV infections may be explained by a higher affinity of spike protein for ACE2. Entry of the virus requires cleavage of spike protein, which is dependent on the proteases available in different cell types. It has been demonstrated that there is an involvement of the cellular serine protease TMPRSS2 (transmembrane protein serine protease 2) and endosomal cathepsins in the virus entry (Xu *et al.*, 2020). After fusion, the envelope and capsid part of the virus are removed and its genetic material is released into the host cell. The viral genome takes over the host cell machinery and guides the synthesis of its proteins and genetic material. Chymotrypsin-like protease (3CLpro) helps in slicing of polypeptides for the production of functional proteins. Viral particles are assembled and newly synthesised virions leave the cells through exocytosis and infect other cells (Lu *et al.*, 2020; Xu *et al.*, 2020; Zhu *et al.*, 2020).

Functional food plants with immunomodulatory and antiviral properties

It has long been observed that diet and health have many links. Recent studies have proven that certain foods or nutraceutical products may help in preventing the spread of the disease. Therefore, an interest in functional foods and dietary supplements have increased during this COVID time and people have started incorporating them in their daily diet. Several foods have shown to contain compounds, which can enhance our immune system to fight against the infection or can eliminate the pathogen through their antiviral activity. Garlic have shown to strengthen our immune system, as well as have antiviral properties (Clement *et al.*, 2010; Thuy *et al.*, 2020). Similarly ginger has also shown to block viruses from attaching to cells and is used to treat respiratory infections (Chang *et al.*, 2013). Herbs like tulsi, fenugreek, thyme, oregano have anti-viral and immunomodulatory properties (Yasmin *et al.*, 2020). Cruciferous vegetables such as broccoli, cauliflower and cabbage have also shown to improve our immune system against the viral infection (Tsai *et al.*, 2010). Leafy greens, such as spinach, kale are packed with nutrients, which have been found to stimulate the immune system beyond the nutritional benefits (Mensah *et al.,* 2008). Nuts and seeds help the body to produce T-cells, which in turn can kill off infectious particles (Wu *et al.,* 2018). Citurs foods such as amla, lemon, oranges, red peppers, also help to fight against infection by boosting our immune system (Singh *et al.,* 2020).

Licorice, an extract from the root of the plant *Glycyrrhiza glabra* has been consumed by humans since ancient times and is used as a flavouring agent as well as health supplement. The root contains compounds, which are responsible for immunomodulation, antiviral and other biological activities (Damle, 2014). Licorice when tested on SARS-CoV-infected patients showed inhibition of SARS-CoV replication (Cinat *et al.,* 2003). Research found that cranberry juice and pomegranate juice have the potential to kill the SARS-CoV-2 virus (Conzelmann, 2020). Extract of dried bark of Cinnamon was found to inhibit SARS-CoV infection (Zhuang *et al.,* 2009). Researchers have claimed that chemical compounds present in cocoa and dark chocolate, can block a particular protease of SARS-CoV-2, thereby preventing the infection (Zhu and Xie, 2020). Black tea and green tea decoction showed activation of cell-mediated immunity and an increase in lymphoproliferative action, they stimulate T-cells, which are responsible for killing pathogens such as viruses and bacteria that evade our body (Chattopadhyay *et al.,* 2021; Zhu and Xie, 2020). Citrus and galangal constituents have been tested against SARS-CoV-2 and have shown possibility to fight the infection (Utomo and Meiyanto, 2020). Extracts of mango leaves have shown to enhance antibody levels, increase in WBC count and the size of the thymus and spleen (Al-Rawi *et al.,* 2019). *Nigella sativa* extracts have demonstrated its inhibitory activity against certain viral pathogens (Ahmad *et al.,* 2013).

Important phytonutrients affective against Coronavirus

Polyphenols

Polyphenols are the largest class of bioactive compounds present in plants, which are produced as secondary metabolites with protective functions against biotic and abiotic stresses. Structurally, the term polyphenol refers to the presence of one or more phenolic rings with hydroxyl groups. Polyphenols can be classified into phenolic acids (e.g. cinnamic acid, ferulic acid, caeffic acid etc), flavonoids (including anthocyanins, flavones, flavanones, flavonols, is of lavones, and flavan-3-ols), polyphenolic amides, and other polyphenol compounds, such as stilbines, ligansetc (Yahfoufi *et al.,* 2018). Besides the well-known antioxidant and anti-inflammatory activities of polyphenols, evidence suggest antiviral activity of these class of compounds against several viruses, such as herpes simplex virus (HSV), influenza virus, Epstein-Barr virus (Ding *et al.,* 2018). Recent evidences have demonstrated activity against coronavirus, thereby increasing interest against these class of phytochemicals.

It was recently suggested that dietary intake of resveratrol, a polyphenol found at high concentrations in the skin of red wine grapes (Vitis vinifera) blueberries, cranberries, strawberries, peanuts, pistachios could modulate SARS-CoV-2 disease severity by regulating ACE2 expression and function (Horne and Vohl, 2020). Flavanols and proanthocyanidins present in dark chocolate, green tea and grapes have shown to block the activity of the main protease required for the virus to replicate and assemble itself in the virus (Ghosh *et al.,* 2020; Yue and Xie, 2020). Catechins in tea are also antimicrobial, antioxidative, and may help reduce disease risk (Jena *et al.,* 2020). The immunosti-mulatory properties of black tea and green tea are due to the presence of (–)-epigallocatechin gallate, quercetin and gallic acid in the leaves (Ghosh *et al.,* 2020).

Curcumin a polyphenol found in the turmeric has shown excellent antiviral properties against various viral diseases. With all the antiviral properties curcumin shows antihistaminic, anti-inflammatory, and bronchodilator effects thereby relieving the respiratory troubles caused by a coronavirus (Manoharan *et al.,* 2020). It also strengthens the immune system to fight against the infection (Catanzaro *et al.,* 2018). Curcumin can interact with several types of immune cells, including dendritic cells, B- and T-lymphocytes, macrophages and inflammatory cytokines and enhance the defence mechanism of the host (Catanzaro *et al.,* 2018; Jena *et al.,* 2020). Luteolin and quercetin, another important polyphenols found in various fruits and vegetables have shown to inhibited SARS-CoV infection by preventing virus entry into the cells by binding with spike protein of the virus (Schettig *et al.,* 2020). Emodin, an anthraquinone-type polyphenol found in rhubarb, a vegetable derived from *Rheum officinale* also binds with spike protein, thereby interfering in its interaction with the receptor (Ho *et al.,* 2007). Naringenin, found in a variety of herbs and fruits, had also shown a stronger binding affinity with the spike protein (Ubani *et al.,* 2020). Dietary flavonoids such as kaempferol and quercetin were shown to inhibit SARS-CoV serine protease3CLpro in an in vitro study (Park *et al.,* 2017). Quercetin and kaempferol also inhibited RNA dependent RNA polymerase enzyme, which is necessary for the virus to replicate (Singh *et al.,* 2020).

These polyphenols, such as curcumin, resveratrol, kaempferol etc have also shown to reduce the damaging effects of cytokine storm associated with coronavirus infection (Yahfoufi *et al.,* 2018). Cytokine storm is a condition when our own immune system instead of fighting with the infection, goes rogue, creating more havoc than the disease itself. High levels of inflammation is produced, sometimes it can be fatal (Yahfoufi *et al.,* 2018). This type of condition is responsible for the intense illnesses some people are experiencing.

Vitamins

Vitamins play a vital role in both innate and adaptive immune responses and are required by the body to fight against infection (Gombart *et al.,* 2020). Vitamin C is a water-soluble vitamin that is present in a variety of fruits and vegetables, such as amla, oranges, lemon, bell peppers etc. and is responsible for various physiological function of the body. It is essential for the growth and repair of tissue and help in supporting a healthy immune system (Carr and Maggini, 2017). Reports are available where Vitamin C had been successfully used for the treatment of moderate to severe cases of COVID-19 (Alan *et al.,* 2020). Vitamin C along with other vitamins when given to infected individuals was found to inhibit the spread of SARS- CoV-2 infection (Banerjee, 2020). Vitamin C may prevent the severity of lower respiratory tract problems arising due to the disease and had been given in combination with other medication to treat COVID patients (Carr, 2020). Vitamin D, a group of lipid-soluble micronutrients, is obtained either by exposure to UVB radiation or from some food sources, such as eggs, fish, mushroom etc. Vitamin D has an important role in innate and adaptive immune responses and it is observed that its deficiency is associated with increased autoimmunity as well as an increased susceptibility to infection (Fabbri *et al.,* 2020). Vitamin D deficiency is the most common risk factor for critically ill COVID-19 patients. Several studies have stated the likely relationship between COVID-19 mortality and vitamin D deficiency (Alipio, 2020). It has been reported that Vitamin D could induce the release of antimicrobial peptides which can reduce SARS-CoV-2 replication and downregulate pro-inflammatory cytokines (Ghavideldarestani *et al.,* 2020). It has been found that Vitamin D binds with angiotensin-converting enzyme 2 (ACE2) receptor and prevent virus particles from binding, thus inhibiting spread of the infection (Ilie *et al.,* 2020). Vitamin B plays an important role in proper cell functioning, energy metabolism and modulation of innate and adaptive immune responses. B vitamins can be found in a variety of foods including red meat, beans, milk, cheese, broccoli, spinach, avocados and brown rice (Yoshii *et al.,* 2019). It has been observed that Vitamin B helps COVID patients by reducing pro-inflammatory cytokine levels and improving respiratory problems associated with the disease (Carella *et al.,* 2020). Vitamin B-12 is one of the many B vitamins that are crucial for bodily health. The most profound benefit of B-12 is its ability to regulate cell metabolism and boost red blood cells production. Many studies have linked Vitamin B-12 deficiency to severe COVID-19 cases. Researchers suggested that COVID-19 can stop RBC formation in the body, and lack of vitamin B-12 could make it worse (Lopes, 2020). Researchers found that loss of erythrocytes in Coronavirus patients could damage brain neurons, blood vessels, and lead to multiple organ failure in worse cases (Mary *et al.,* 2020). Vitamin E, is a lipid-soluble compound, found in higher concentration in immune cells is known to modulate immune function, particularly T cell function by controlling membrane integrity, signal transduction, and cell division. Its deficiency has been observed to impair normal functions of the immune system and increase in pathogenicity of disease (Lee and Han, 2018). Vitamin E has also shown to reduce risk of respiratory tract infection (Graat *et al.,* 2002).

Trace element

Selenium (Se) is an essential trace element that occurs as selenocysteine in catalytical centers of many selenoproteins and play critical roles in various biological functions (Hoffmann and Berry, 2008). It has been observed that Se deficiency is associated with immune system dysfunction and also with several viral and bacterial infections. (Hiffler, 2020). It has been shown that critically ill patients suffering from viral diseases had a rapid drop in Se level and dietary intake of Se has improved recovery of patient suffering from viral disease (Hoffmann and Berry, 2008). In this current COVID time focus is made to provide adequate amount of Se to lower the pathogenicity of virus. It has been observed that a Se dependent enzyme, glutathione peroxidase1 interacts with a main protease of SARS-CoV-2 responsible for the viral replication, thereby inhibiting its propagation (Lucia *et al.,* 2020).

Zinc is a mineral found in many different food types. Foods high in zinc include animal products, such as meat, shellfish, chicken, and fortified breakfast cereal, beans, nuts, and seeds. Zinc is crucial for many biological processes and is required for the proper function of the nervous and the cardiovascular systems. Zinc homeostasis has a critical role in the maintenance of adaptive and innate immunity (Chasapis *et al.,* 2011). Zinc is a component of many enzymes, proteases, and polymerase and exerts its functions as a signaling molecule and a metal cofactor needed by several enzymes for proper function of the immune system (Maywald *et al.,* 2017). Recent studies have focused on the benefits of zinc against COVID-19. The findings suggest that Zinc, with its potential antiviral properties could have protective effects against COVID-19 (Read *et al.,* 2019). An in vitro experimental study has shown that chloroquine, which was used as a treatment option early on in the pandemic has antiviral activity against SARS-CoV-2 (Colson *et al.,* 2020). Chloroquine, as ionophore of zinc, increases zinc flux into the cells, thereby causing a decrease in the severity of infection (Xue *et al.,* 2014). A study showed that when doctors treated patients with zinc and hydroxychloroquine, they discharged more patients, and fewer people died from COVID-19 (Colson *et al.,* 2020).

References

1. Ahmad, A., Husain, A., Mujeeb, M., Khan, S. A., Najmi, A. K., Siddique, N. A. *et al.* 2013. A review on therapeutic potential of Nigella sativa: A miracle herb. Asian Pac J Trop Biomed. 3: 337–352.
2. Alan Rossetti, C., Pablo Real, J., Daniel Palma, S., 2020. High dose of ascorbic acid used insars Covid-19 treatment: scientific and clinical support for its therapeutic implementation. Ars Pharm. 61: 145–148.
3. Alipio, M., 2020. Vitamin D supplementation could possibly improve clinical outcomes of patients infected with coronavirus-2019 (COVID-2019). SSRN Electron J. doi:https:// doi.org/10.2139/ssrn.3571484.
4. Al-Rawi, A. A. S., Al-Dulaimi, H. S. H., Al-Rawi, M. A. A. 2019. Antiviral Activity of Mangifera Extract on Influenza Virus Cultivated in Different Cell Cultures. J Pure Appl Microbiol. 13: 455–458.
5. Banerjee, S., 2020. Safety & Efficacy of established medicine in controlling COVID-19 SARS-CoV2 infection in a home-quarantine environment. Preprint doi: 10.13140/RG.2.2.24554.67526/3.
6. Bohn, M.K., Hall, A., Sepiashvili, L., Jung, B., Steele, S., Adeli, K. 2020. Pathophysiology of COVID-19: Mechanisms Underlying Disease Severity and Progression. Physiol. 35: 288–301.
7. Brian, D.A., Baric, R.S. 2005. Coronavirus genome structure and replication. Curr Top Microbiol Immunol. 287: 1–30.
8. Carella, A.M., Benvenuto, A., Lagattolla, V., Marinelli, T., De Luca, P., Ciavarrella, G. 2020. Vitamin supplements in the Era of SARS-Cov2 pandemic. GSCBPS. 11: 07-19.
9. Carr, A., Maggini, S. 2017. Vitamin C and immune function. Nutrients. doi: 10.3390/nu9111211.
10. Carr, A.C., 2020. A new clinical trial to test high-dose vitamin C in patients with COVID-19. Crit Care. 24: 1–2.
11. Catanzaro, M., Corsini, E., Rosini, M., Racchi, M., Lanni, C. 2018. Immunomodulators inspired by nature: A review on Curcumin and Echinacea. Molecules. 23: 27–78.

12. Chafekar, A., Fielding, B. C. 2018. MERS-CoV: Understanding the latest human coronavirus threat. Viruses. 10: 93-115.

13. Chang, J.S., Wang, K.C., Yeh, C.F., Shieh, D.E., Chiang, L.C. 2013. Fresh ginger (Zingiber officinale) has anti-viral activity against human respiratory syncytial virus in human respiratory tract cell lines. J Ethnopharmacol. 145: 146-51.

14. Chasapis, C.T., Loutsidou, A.C., Spiliopoulou, C.A., Stefanidou, M.E. 2012. Zinc and human health: an update. Arch Toxicol. 86: 521–534.

15. Chattopadhyay, C., Chakrabarti, N., Chatterjee, M., Mukherjee, S., Sarkar, K., Chaudhuri, R. 2012. Black tea (Camellia sinensis) decoction shows immunomodulatory properties on an experimental animal model and in human peripheral mononuclear cells. Pharmacognosy Res. 4: 15–21.

16. Chen, N., Zhou, M., Dong, X., Qu, J., Gong, F., Han, Y. *et al.* 2020. Epidemiological and clinical characteristics of 99 cases of 2019 novel coronavirus pneumonia in Wuhan, China: A descriptive study. Lancet, 395: 507–513.

17. Cheng, P. K., Wong, D. A., Tong, L. K., Ip, S. M., Lo, A. C., Lau, C. S. et al. 2004. Viral shedding patterns of coronavirus in patients with probable severe acute respiratory syndrome. Lancet. 363: 1699–1700.

18. Chojnackaa, K., Witek-Krowiaka, A., Skrzypczaka, D., Mikulaa, K., M³ynarzb, P. 2020. Phytochemicals containing biologically active polyphenols as an effective agent against Covid-19-inducing coronavirus. J Funct Foods. 73: 1-8.

19. Cinat, J., Morgenstern, B., Bauer, G., Chandra, P., Rabenau, H., Doerr, H. W. 2003. Glycyrrhizin, an active component of liquorice roots, and replication of SARS- associated coronavirus. Lancet. 361: 2045–2046.

20. Clement, F., Pramod, S. N., Venkatesh, Y. P. 2010. Identity of the immuno-modulatory proteins from garlic (Allium sativum) with the major garlic lectins or agglutinins. Int Immunopharmacol. 10: 316–324.

21. Colson, P., Rolain, J.M., Lagier, J.C., Brouqui, P., Raoult, D., 2020. Chloroquine and hydroxychloroquine as available weapons to fight COVID-19. Int J Antimicrob Agents doi:https://doi.org/10.1016/j.ijantimicag.2020.105932 0.

22. Conzelmann, C., Weil, T., Gro, R., Jungke, P., Frank, B., Eggers, M., Müller, J.A., Münch, J. 2020. Antiviral activity of plant juices and green tea against SARS-CoV-2 and influenza virus in vitro. bio Rxiv. doi:https://doi.org/10.1101/2020.10.30.360545.

23. Damle, M. 2014. Glycyrrhiza glabra (Liquorice) - a potent medicinal herb. International J Herb Med. 2: 132–136.

24. Ding, S., Jiang, H., Fang, J. 2018. Regulation of immune function by polyphenols. J Immunol. doi: https://doi.org/10.1155/2018/1264074.

25. Fabbri, A., Infante, M., Ricordi, C., 2020. Editorial–Vitamin D status: a key modulator of innate immunity and natural defense from acute viral respiratory infections. Eur Rev Med Pharmacol Sci. 24: 4048–4052.

26. Ghavideldarestani, M., Honardoost, M., Khamseh, M.E., 2020. Role of vitamin D in pathogenesis and severity of COVID-19 infection. Preprints. doi: 10.1080/13813455.2020.1792505

27. Ghosh, R., Chakraborty, A., Biswas, A., Chowdhuri, S. 2020. Evaluation of green tea polyphenols as novel corona virus (SARS CoV-2) main protease (Mpro)

inhibitors – an in silico docking and molecular dynamics simulation study. J Biomol. doi: 10.1080/07391102.2020.1779818.

28. Gombart, A.F., Pierre, A., Maggini, S. 2020. A review of micronutrients and the immune System–Working in harmony to reduce the risk of infection. Nutrients 12: 236-277.
29. Graat, J.M., Schouten, E.G., Kok, F.J. 2002. Effect of daily vitamin E and multivitamin- mineral supplementation on acute respiratory tract infections in elderly persons: a randomized controlled trial. JAMA. 288: 715–21.
30. Hiffler, L., 2020. Selenium and RNA viruses interactions: potential implications for SARSCov-2 infection (Covid-19). Front Nutr. doi. https://doi.org/10.3389/fnut.2020.00164.
31. Ho, T.Y., Wu, S.L., Chen, J.C., Li, C.C., Hsiang, C.Y. 2007. Emodin blocks the SARS coronavirus spike protein and angiotensin-converting enzyme 2 interaction. Antivir Res. 74: 92-101.
32. Hoffmann, P.R., Berry, M.J., 2008. The influence of selenium on immune responses. Mol Nutr Food Res. 52: 1273–1280.
33. Hornem, J, R., Vohl, M.C. 2020. Biological plausibility for interactions between dietary fat, resveratrol, ACE2, and SARS-CoV illness severity. Am J Physiol Endocrinol Metab. 318: 830-833.
34. Huang, C., Wang, Y., Li, X., Ren, L., Zhao, J., Hu, Y. *et al.* 2020. Clinical features of patients infected with 2019 novel coronavirus in Wuhan, China. Lancet. 395: 497–506.
35. Ilie, P., Stefanescu, S., Smith, L., 2020. The role of Vitamin D in the prevention of Coronavirus Disease 2019 infection and mortality. Aging Clin Exp Res. 32: 1195–1198.
36. Islam, M.T., Sarkar, C., El-Kersh, D.M., Jamaddar, S., Uddin, S.J., Shilpi, J.A., Mubarak,M.S. 2020. Natural products and their derivatives against coronavirus: A review of the non-clinical and pre-clinical data. Phytother Res. 34: 2471–2492.
37. Jena, A.B., Kanungo, N., Nayak, V., Chainy, G., Dandapat, J. 2020. Catechin and Curcumin interact with corona (2019-nCoV/SARS-CoV2) viral S protein and ACE2 of human cell membrane: insights from computational study and implication for intervention. Preprint from Research Square. doi. http://dx.doi.org/10.21203/ rs.3.rs-22057/v1.
38. Lee, G., Han, S. 2018. The role of vitamin E in immunity. Nutrients. doi: https://doi.org/10.3390/nu10111614.
39. Lopes, M.J.S. 2020. Can vitamin B12 be an adjuvant to COVID-19 treatment? GSCBPS. 11: 01-05
40. Lu, R., Zhao, X., Li, J., Niu, P., Yang, B., Wu, H., *et al.* 2020. Genomic characterisationand epidemiology of 2019 novel coronavirus: implications for virus origins and receptor binding. Lancet. 395: 565–74.
41. Manoharan, Y., Haridas, V., Vasanthakumar, K.C., Muthu, S., Thavoorullah, F.F., Shetty, P. 2020. Curcumin: a wonder drug as a preventive measure for COVID-19 management. Ind J Clin Biochem. 35: 373-375.

42. Maywald, M., Wessels, I., Rink, L. 2017. Zinc signals and immunity. Int J Mol Sci doi:10.3390/ijms18102222.
43. Mensah, J.K., Okoli, R.I., Ohaju-Obodo, J.O., Eifediyi, K. 2008. Phytochemical, nutritional and medical properties of some leafy vegetables consumed by Edo people of Nigeria. Afr J Biotechnol. 7: 2304-2309.
44. Park, J.Y., Yuk, H.J., Ryu, H.W., Lim, S.H., Kim, K.S., Park, K.H. *et al.* 2017. Evaluation of polyphenols from Broussonetiapapyrifera as coronavirus protease inhibitors. J Enzyme Inhib Med Chem. 32:504-512.
45. Pedersen, S.F., Ho, Y.C. 2020. SARS-CoV-2: a storm is raging. J Clin Invest. 130:2202–2205.
46. Read, S.A., Obeid, S., Ahlenstiel, C., Ahlenstiel, G. 2019. The role of zinc in antiviral immunity. Adv Nutr. 10:696–710.
47. Sahebnasagh, A., Saghafi, F., Avan, R., Khoshi, A., Khataminia, M., Safdari, M., Habtemariam, S., Ghaleno, H.R., Nabavi, S.M. 2020. The prophylaxis and treatment potential of supplements for COVID-19. Eur J Pharmacol. 887: 1-11.
48. Schettig, R., Sears, T., Klein, M., Tan-Lim, R., Matthias Jr, R., Aussems, *et al.* 2020. COVID-19 patient with multifocal pneumonia and respiratory difficulty resolved quickly: possible antiviral and anti-inflammatory benefits of Quercinex (Nebulized Quercetin-NAC) as adjuvant. Ther Adv Infect Dis. 10: 45-55.
49. Seale, L.A., Torres, D.J., Berry, M.J., Pitts, M.W. 2020. A role for selenium-dependent GPX1 in SARS-CoV-2 virulence. Am J Clin Nutr. 112: 447–448.
50. Singh, B., Singh, J.P., Kaur, A., Singh, N. 2020. Phenolic composition, antioxidant potential and health benefits of citrus peel. Food Res Int. 132: 109-114.
51. Singh, S., Sonawane, A., Sadhukhan, S. 2020. Plant-derived natural polyphenols as potential antiviral drugs against SARS-CoV-2 via RNA-dependent RNA polymerase (RdRp) inhibition: an in-silico analysis. J Biomol. doi: 10.1080/07391102.2020.1796810.
52. Thuy, B.T.P., My, T.T.A., Hai, N.T.T., Hieu, L.T., Hoa, T.T., Thi, Phuong Loan H, *et al.* 2020. Investigation into SARS-CoV-2 resistance of compounds in garlic essential oil. ACS Omega. 5: 8312–8320.
53. Tsai, J., Liu, H., Chen, Y. 2010. Suppression of Inflammatory Mediators by Cruciferous Vegetable-Derived Indole-3-Carbinol and Phenylethyl Isothiocyanate in Lipopolysaccharide-Activated Macrophages. Mediators Inflamm. 2010: 1-5.
54. Ubani, A., Agwom, F., Morenikeji, O.R., Shehu, N.Y., Luka, P., Umera, E.A., Umar, U., Omale, S., Nnadi, E., Aguiyi, J.C. 2020. Molecular docking analysis of some phytochemicals on two SARS-CoV-2 targets. BioRxiv. doi: http://dx.doi.org/10.1101/2020.03.31.017657. 03.31.017657.
55. Utomo, R.Y., Meiyanto, E. 2020. Revealing the potency of citrus and galangal constituents to halt SARS-CoV-2 infection. Preprints. doi. http://dx.doi.org/10.20944.
56. Worldometer, 2020. Coronavirus. https://www.worldometers.info/coronavirus.
57. Wu, D., Lewis, E.D., Pae, M., Meydani, S.N. 2018. Nutritional Modulation of Immune Function: Analysis of Evidence, Mechanisms, and Clinical Relevance. Front Immunol. 9: 1-19.

58. Xu, X., Chen, P., Wang, J., Feng, J., Zhou, H., Li, X. *et al.* 2020. Evolution of the novel coronavirus from the ongoing Wuhan outbreak and modeling of its spike protein for risk of human transmission. Science China. Life Sci. 63: 457–460.

59. Xue, J., Moyer, A., Peng, B., Wu, J., Hannafon, B.N., Ding, W.-Q., 2014. Chloroquine is a zinc ionophore. PLOS one. 9: 1-6.

60. Yahfoufi, N., Alsadi, N., Jambi, M., Matar, C. 2018. The immunomodulatory and anti-inflammatory role of polyphenols. Nutrients. 10:1-23.

61. Yasmin, A.R., Chia, S.L., .Looi, Q.H., Omar, A.R., Noordin, M.M., Ideris, A. 2020. Herbal extracts as antiviral agents. In, Feed Additives, Aromatic Plants and Herbs in Animal Nutrition and Health. Pages 115-132.

62. Yoshii, K., Hosomi, K., Sawane, K., Kunisawa, J. 2019. Metabolism of dietary and microbial vitamin B family in the regulation of host immunity. Front Nutr. 6:1-12.

63. Zhu, N., Zhang, D., Wang, W., Li, X., Yang, B., Song, J. *et al.* 2020. A novel coronavirus from patients with pneumonia in China, 2019. New Engl J Med. 382: 727–733.

64. Zhu, Y., Xie, D. 2020. Docking characterization and in vitro inhibitory activity of flavan-3-ols and dimeric proanthocyanidins against the main protease activity of SARS-Cov-2. Front. Plant Sci. doi: 10.3389/fpls.2020.601316

65. Zhuang, M., Jiang, H., Suzuki, Y., Li, X., Xiao, P., Tanaka. *et al.* 2009. Procyanidins and butanol extract of Cinnamomi Cortex inhibit SARS-CoV infection. Antiviral Res. 82: 73–81.

7

Synbiotic Foods: A Boon to Human Health

Dr Reena Verma, Dr Gargi Saxena

The modern-day sedentary lifestyle and eating patterns have diminished the immunity of an individual, which is further worsened by the COVID-19 infection which is spreading at a wide pace. Entire mankind across the globe is suffering in the wake of the COVID-19 outbreak which calls for the maintenance and enhancement of immunity. Since balance of bacteria in our gut influences the balance of our immune system, the incorporation of functional probiotics in the daily diet is vital for boosting immunity.

Synbiotics are the right choice to meet the need of an hour, as they play an essential role in reducing the symptoms of the COVID-19 *i.e.,* respiratory and digestive problems. Synergistic products are the combination of pro and prebiotics, which helps in maintaining the gut health of the organism by enhancing the survival and implantation of live microbial food additives in the gastrointestinal tract, thereby stimulating growth and causing the metabolism of health-promoting bacteria, thus improving the health of host.

In recent years, there have been advances in the fermented food product industry in context to the microbes and fermentable polysaccharides used for their production, for better health effects. The application of microbial strains of *Lactobacillus, Bifidobacterium* and *Saccharomyces* is booming presently in fermentation industry dealing with dairy and non- dairy substrates. The non-dairy substrates like cereals, pseudo-cereals, legumes, nuts and seeds were considered as the promising source to overcome the limitations imposed by milk-based products like lactose intolerance and cholesterol content. Furthermore, the addition of prebiotics as chicory root, almonds, pectin, onion, leeks etc. enhances the growth of probiotics in the intestines, leading to improved gut health and thus boosts immunity to fight against the deadly infection.

Modern Diet and its Impact on Human Health

The famous quote from Hippocrates **"Let food be thy medicine"** appreciates and explains the direct relationship between health and nutrition since antiquity. But it was true in the earlier times as the use of chemical fertilisers and pesticides were low or negligible, the water used for irrigation was also safe for human consumption, the population was also less leading to better food security and better standard of living. Increase in population has increased the demand of food which in turn has led to the advances in food production technologies like genetically engineered foods, formulation of processed and semi-processed foods and increased usage of chemical fertilisers and pesticides, which have adverse effects on the overall health of the population. Besides all these factors, sedentary lifestyle, imbalanced diets and lack of exercise have also contributed to the prevalence of non-communicable diseases. The situation is becoming more unfavourable due to the privatisation of jobs, with hectic work schedules and odd working hours disturbing the biological clocks, which in turn leads to the dramatic reduction in people's exercising pattern. Lack of exercise, besides influencing the metabolism, also appears to profoundly shape immune responses, which is further worsened by pandemic caused by the COVID-19 virus.

Eating enough nutrients as part of a balanced diet is required for the health and function of all cells, including immune cells, to maintain a good standard of life and longevity.

To prepare the body to combat microbial attacks and excess inflammation, certain dietary patterns should be followed, but it should not be confused with the idea that individual foods can offer special protection because each stage of the immune response relies on the presence of many micronutrients in the human body. The important nutrients that are required for the growth and function of immune cells are vitamin C, vitamin D, zinc, selenium, iron, and protein, including the amino acid glutamine. Many plant and animal foods are good sources of these nutrients, so regular consumption of nutritious diet can build up the immune system.

Food always relates to health and nutrition but we are living in the era where relating food as the only factor for health and nutrition is less justified. Following a diet that is limited in variety and low in nutrients, both qualitatively and quantitatively, can negatively affect a healthy immune system. The example of such diets are the diets primarily consisting of ultra-processed foods, high in sodium and sugar, canned and ready-to-eat meals. It is also believed that a diet high in refined sugar and trans fats and low in fruits and vegetables can 3 promote disturbances in healthy intestinal microorganisms, resulting in chronic inflammation of the gut, and associated suppressed immunity.

The Concept

Several species of bacteria lives in lumen of human colon. Colon' refers to colony or microbiota colonisation, that plays significant role in prebiotic fermentation. Present-day prebiotic outlook is well established in several clinical trials conducted on animals and humans for attenuating gut dysbiosis. However, the attempt to connect the dots between the bacterial population and the host is not easily discernible due to the huge amount of gut microbiome. So, the need to examine recent work on prebiotic metabolism pathways accepted by widely studied probiotics i.e., *Lactobacillus* and *bifidobacteria*.

Awareness and tendency of global consumers for balanced dietary items capable of granting health benefits in addition to supplying basic nutrition led to the evolving concept of functional foods. Foods which contain some component(s) that promote health beyond traditional nutrients are called functional foods. Proven clinical evidence has projected probiotics as one of the fastest rising functional food categories. The hunt for analysing the importance of a wide variety of food components and nutrients in improving health and aiding in prevention of chronic diseases continues. Research shows a range of new food types that have demonstrated distinct advantages and are called functional foods.

Functional food concept emphasises that food is not only crucial to health; it also plays a role not in the prevention of diseases but in lessening of risk factors for many diseases. It also improves certain essential physiological functions. Functional foods are rich in required amount of vitamins, fats, proteins, carbohydrates and hence are evolving rapidly.

Probiotics

Fermentation of foods is an age old method used for the preservation of food. Fermentation process is done by the addition of bacterial or yeast cultures like lactic acid bacteria (LAB) and fungi respectively. The traditional fermented foods are the potential source of microorganisms and show probiotic characteristics. Fermented products are rich in Vitamin C content, have better bioavailability of protein and are easily digestible also. There is an increase in the bioavailability of minerals like phosphorous, iron and zinc due to the action of microbial enzymes such as phytases, or due to the organic acids produced during fermentation of cereals. Focussing on the present day scenario, there is an alleviation in the development of non-dairy based fermented foods instead of diary based fermented foods. Fruit and vegetable based, cereals based and soya based foods are gaining importance among the non-dairy based fermented foods.

Concept and Definition

The original probiotic term is "*Probiotika*" derived from Latin word which where "pro" means favour, and the Greek word "bios" which means life. In 2001, FAO/WHO formulated our current concept of probiotics as "live microorganisms that, when administered in sufficient quantities, confer health benefits to the host." Probiotics are commonly described as live microorganisms, ideally of human origin, which yield unspecified health benefits on the host upon ingestion in appropriate amounts. The therapeutic effect of probiotic bacteria has been assessed many fundamental, experimental and in-clinic studies over years. These are distributed particularly in the gastrointestinal tract to improve microbiota composition. These consist of *Saccharomyces boulardii* leaven or lactic acid bacteria, such as the species *Lactobacillus* and *Bifidobacterium*, and are regulated in the form of dietary supplements and foods.

The water activity, processing and storage temperature, shelf life, oxygen content, pH, mechanical stress, salt content, and content of other harmful or essential ingredients are the general factors that affects the applicability of probiotics in food products. Excess water activity is a critical parameter that increases the death rate of bacteria in many products, for example, cereals, chocolate, marmalade, honey, and toffees because these products are too "dry" for applying live bacteria and too "wet" for the application of freeze-dried bacteria. Freeze-dried bacteria could be applied in these products if the bacteria could be protected from moisture, as small amounts of moisture can be very detrimental to the dried culture.

In addition to dairy products, fruit juices have been shown to be suitable carriers for probiotics wherein the limiting factor for many of the probiotic strains is the low pH of the juices. There is growing interest in consumers towards healthier foods and probiotic juices from sources liked fruits and vegetables, and cereal and pulse based beverages that can serve as an healthier beverage option. But, the application of probiotic cultures in non-dairy products and environments represents a great challenge and needs to be researched at the industrial level for commercial production of these healthy products.

Probiotics demonstrate many ways of action: antagonism to pathogenic bacteria by production of products that inhibit their growth, such as bacteriocins, organic acids and hydrogen peroxide; or competing for locations adhering to the mucous membranes of the intestines; or competition for nutrients.

Characteristics of Ideal Probiotic organisms

There is a rise in food production enriched with active ingredients such as prebiotics, probiotics and synbiotics that are known as functional food. Probiotics are commonly used as food supplements because of clinical evidence that supports the idea that maintaining a balanced gut microflora protects against gastrointestinal disorder including infection and inflammatory bowel syndromes.

Healthy probiotic should be non-pathogenic. Also, it should be non-toxic and sufficiently competent to enhance beneficial effects on the applied host. They must produce antimicrobial compounds (hydrogen peroxide, organic acids, bacteriocins and siderophores), sustain and metabolise in the intestine, bile salts, organic acids, and proteases at low pH. They should also enhance the immune response and be able to exercise at least one scientifically proven health enhancing feature/quality to the applied host.

Along with the above stated qualities, Probiotics should bear a good shelf life and should be able to reinstate and replace the intestinal micro flora. The effective probiotic cell numbers in a drug should be at least 106 CFU/mL at the safety and functional claim date of expiry, as the suggested minimum effective dose per day should be around 110 cells.

Probiotic Microorganisms

The factors related to a microorganisms workable cell count in a product in the entire manufacturing process and period of shelf-life are low pH, acidity, packaging conditions, redox potential, hydrogen peroxide, flavouring agents, packaging materials etc. Probiotic micro-organisms most widely used against pathogens are Lactobacillus acidophilus, *Lactobacillus rhamnosusGG, Saccharomyces boulardii, Bifidobacterium bifidum* and *Bacillus coagulans*. The use of *Lactobacilli* and further probiotics in combination with antibiotics too seems encouraging for the treatment of diseases caused by bacteria, but further well-designed precise trials with standard methodologies and bigger size trials are required to prove conclusive benefits.

There are more than 50 species of *lacbtobacilli*, approximately 30 species of *bifidobacteria*, *Saccaromyces*- the only yeast probiotic, *Streptococcus*, *Enterococcus*, *Leuconostoc* etc. The following table shows the major probiotic microorganism candidates used for various purposes.

Lists of Probiotic Candidates

Microorganism	***Genus***	***Species***
Bacteria	*Lactobacillus*	*L. acidophilus*
		L. brevis
		L. reuteri
		L. casei
		L. rhamnosum
		L. bulgaricus
		L. cellobiosus
		L. delbrueckii
		L. fermentum
	Bifidobacterium	*B. thermophilus*
		B. infantis
		B. longum
		B. bifidum
		B. animalis
	Streptococcus	*S. lactis*
		S. thermophilus
		S. cremonis
		S. alivarius
	Bacillus	*B. cagulansPedicoccus*
		P. acidilactici Leuconostoc
		L. mesenteroides
	Enterobacter	*E. faecium*
		E. faecalis
	Saccharomyces	*S. boulardi*
	Lactococcus	*L. lactis subsp. lactis*
	Enterococcus	*E. durans*
	Escherichia	*E. faecium*
		E. coli Nissle

Probiotic Products

The various probiotics classified according to origin are-

- **Dairy-Origin:** Milk, Buttermilk, Yogurt, cheese, ice-cream, fermented milk etc.

  Examples of dairy products are curd, sour cream, buttermilk, bread, and cheese where microbes act as indispensable material for their production and are rich in probiotics.

- **Non-Dairy Origin:** Major non-dairy products comes under the combinations of foods like Cereals and Soy (Bread, Bakery Products, Puddings, Cereal Beverages), Fruits and Vegetables (Juices, Puree, Pulp, Beverages, Dried fruits), Meat and Fish (Sausages).

Health Benefits

Probiotics can play a beneficial role in a variety of medical conditions, including diarrhoea, gastroenteritis, irritable bowel syndrome, inflammatory intestinal disease, hepatic diseases, immune function, child allergies, failure-to-thrive, gut immune homeostasis, hyperlipidaemia, helicobacter pylori based infections etc., all of which have been suggested by some studies to enhance the usage of probiotics. These helps in reducing the health risks factors.

It is not the recent time humanity has experienced the boons of probiotics but benefits of probiotics were already been realised in the past years also. Probiotics are widely recognised for their significance in human and animal nutrition.

PREBIOTICS

Concept and Definition

Prebiotic is described as a substrate selectively used by host micro-organisms that confer a health benefit. These are compounds that encourage the growth or development of beneficial micro-organisms like bacteria and fungi in food. Dietary prebiotics are usually non-digestible fibre compounds which goes through gastrointestinal tract undigested via upper portion and trigger the activity of beneficial bacteria that colonise the large intestine by being a substratum for them.

Prebiotics fermented substrates that exclusively stimulates microflora growth in the gastrointestinal tract and therefore improve host production, composition and activity health.

Fructo-oligosaccharides, inulin, oligo-fructose, lactulose, and galacto-oligosaccharides shows characteristics such as gastric acidity tolerance and mammalian enzymes have been established and fermented by gastrointestinal micro flora, in order to promote further production and growth in beneficial microorganisms selectively. Prebiotic are compounds with intestinal microorganisms that possess intestinal resistance and selective fermentation which includes oligosaccharides, sugar alcohols and polysaccharides. Colonic fermentation is attributed to an intestinal microflora that provides a beneficial effect for humans, including the development of colonprobiosis, increased calcium absorption, increased faecal weight, shorter gastrointestinal transit period and possibly lower blood lipid content. Fermentation is due to the existence of intestinal microflora. The main principle behind is the process of fermentation by which beneficial bacteria in the colon use prebiotics. It has been shown that both Bifidobacteria and Lactobacillus have different prebiotic specificity and that prebiotic fibre is selectively fermented with respect to the bacterial enzymes.

Prebiotics also trigger the increase of harmful and possible pathogenic microbes inside the intestine, in addition to the enhancement of growth of gut bacteria. To be labeled as a prebiotic, it must be shown that prebiotic sources shows benefits on the host. The most well-known example of prebiotics is fermentable carbohydrates derived from fructans and xylans.

Characteristics of Prebiotics

For a compound to be classified as a prebiotic, the following criteria are taken into consideration:

(i) It must be immune to acidic stomach pH, should not be hydrolysed by mammalian enzymes and should show resistance to the gastrointestinal tract absorption.

(ii) May get fermented with the intestinal microbiota.

(iii) This compound can selectively influence the growth and development of the intestinal bacteria which improves health of host.

Types of Prebiotics

Type	*Brief Description*
Fructans	Oligo-fructose or inulin and fructo-oligosaccharide
Galacto-Oligosaccharides	Galacto-oligosaccharides (GOS), a lactose extension product, are categorized into two subgroups as GOS with C3, C4 or C6 excess galactose and GOS derived from lactose through enzymatic transglycosylation.
Starch and Glucose-Derived Oligosaccharides	It is resistant to the upper gut digestion termed as resistant starch (RS) which improves health by producing butyrate more.
Other Oligosaccharides	Certain oligosaccharide originates from a polysaccharide called as pectin. Oligosaccharide of this type is known as pectic oligosaccharide (POS). These are basically based on the galacturonic acid (homogalacturonan) or rhamnose expansion.

(Contd...)

Non-Carbohydrate Oligosaccharides	Though, carbohydrates are likely prebiotic criteria, there exists various compounds which do not comes under the classification of carbohydrates but still are recommended as prebiotics, such as flavonols derived from cocoa

Synbiotics

Synbiotics are the food ingredients or dietary supplements that combine probiotics and prebiotics in a synergistic way, hence termed as synbiotics. Synergistic pro and prebiotic combinations are called synbiotics. The same concept is based on probiotics, prebiotics and synbiotics: the development of foods which multiply bacteria in the intestine after ingestion. However, it is only valid in case of "mutual synergistic" reinforcement. Synbiotics exhibits its benefits in Diarrhoea, Irritable Bowel Syndrome, Inflammatory bowel disorder, Ulcerative colitis and Chrons disease.

Synbiotics incorporates properties of both probiotics and prebiotics and have been known to address some potential problems in gastrointestinal survival of probiotics. A good combination of both pro/prebiotic components in one complete product would therefore ensure a higher impact compared with the pro/prebiotic operation alone. A diet consisting of both the probiotic and prebiotic foods may be more propicious. Probiotic foods contain live helpful bacteria, and prebiotic foods contain fiber and oligosaccharides that feed and maintain healthy colonies of those bacteria. Kefir, yogurt with live active cultures, fermented vegetables, sauerkraut, tempeh, kombucha tea, kimchi, and miso are the examples of probiotic foods whereas prebiotic foods include garlic, onions, leeks, asparagus, Jerusalem artichokes, dandelion greens, bananas, and seaweed. However, daily consumption of a variety of fruits, vegetables, beans, and whole grains for dietary prebiotics can prove to be a general rule to swear by to have a healthier and balanced food plate.

Synbiotics along with other natural foods are now considered essential resources to help sustain good health for humans and animals, for disease prevention and/or as alternatives to mitigate disease-related risks. Studies performed on the human gut and animal gut and immunology microbiota relationship have highlighted the role that synbiotics play in mammalian health. Synbiotics affect the microbial ecology of humans and animals intestines, and play a role in reducing some diseases. They can be the safest and most efficient way to combat colonisation issues especially bacterial pathogens and infection with enteric, pathogens. Functional prebiotic-like foods or natural antimicrobial supplements as alternatives and bioactive metabolite over expression in probiotics are essential for improving synbiotic efficacy.

For human nutrition, following are the popular synbiotic combinations:

- *Lactobacillus*genus bacteria + inulin.
- *Lactobacillus*, *Streptococcus* and *Bifidobacterium* genus bacteria + fructo-oligosaccharides.
- *Lactobacillus, Bifidobacterium, Enterococcus* genus bacteria + fructo-oligosaccharides.
- *Lactobacillus*and *Bifidobacterium* genus bacteria with *oligofructose.*
- *Lactobacillus* and *Bifidobacterium* genus bacteria with inulin.

Mechanism of Synbiotics

Synbiotics acts in two ways:

- By enhanced feasibility of probiotic microorganisms
- By making provision of distinct health effects

The synergistic effect enhances the intestinal metabolic activity, intestinal bio-structure, creation of helpful micro biota and preventing the growth of pathogens inside the gastrointestinal tract. Properties of reducing the levels of metabolites, inhibition of nitrosamines is also observed in synbiotics. It also inhibits carcinogenic stimulants. Their use causes an increase in fatty acids (short-chain), ketones, carbon disulphides and methyl acetates that show a beneficial impact on the health of the host. The following figure helps in understanding the concept and mechanism of synbiotics. Healthy food implies functional food that, in addition to conventional nutritional benefits, has a beneficial impact on more basic body functions. Probiotics along with prebiotics have shown positive health effects, both individually and in a combined form as synbiotics. Hence, the consumers are demanding more such functional foods with good nutritional value, taste, low calories, and therapeutic properties and better shelf life.

Encouraging the Development of Functional Foods

The challenge has just begun to discover novel functional foods, as research provides clear evidence of relationships between dietary components and health benefits. Evaluation of the data for efficacy and safety, insurance of effective regulatory oversight, communicating the

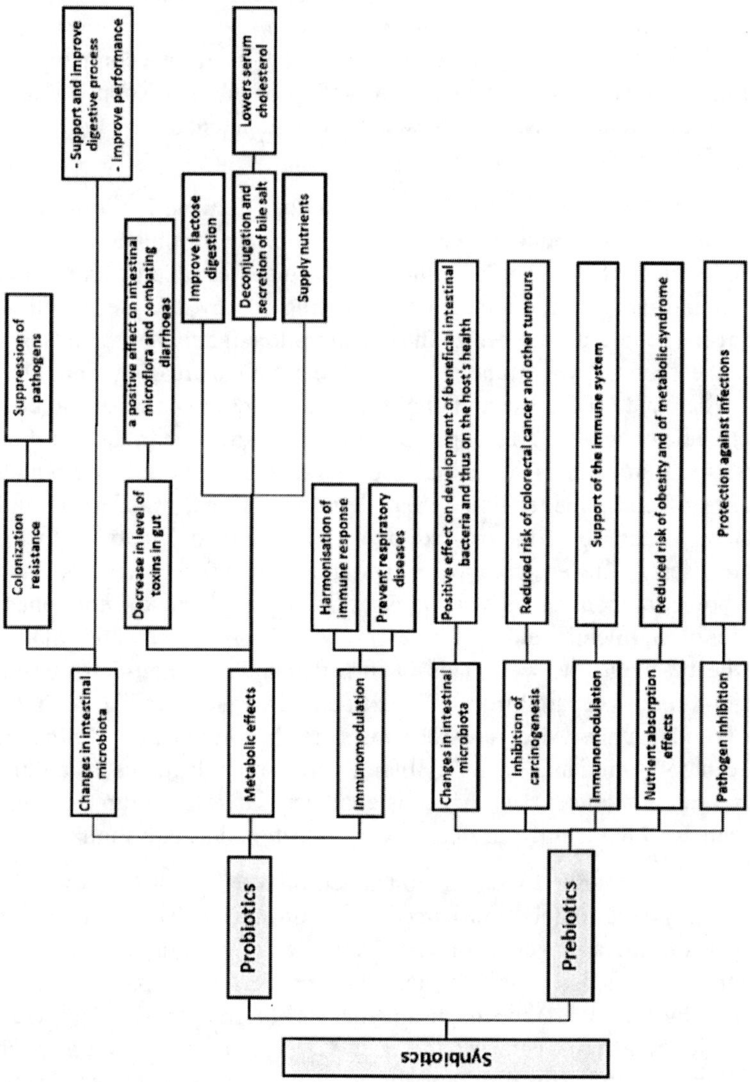

Synbiotics - Concept, Mechanism and Actions

findings to consumers, and providing incentives that encourage research and development of these novel food products requires a scientific, regulatory, and business frameworks to be in place. There should be modifications to the existing efficacy and safety evaluation process to ensure a sound scientific underpinning for each proposed functional food, while providing clear information to consumers, corresponding to the improvements in the regulatory oversight of new functional components. To protect consumer confidence in the safety of the food supply and to encourage the food industry to invest in the development of new functional foods all these changes must be incorporated.

Present day food habits have created a huge demand for consuming no dairy and milk products. The people are looking for milk alternatives as the incidences of obesity, cardiovascular diseases, allergy from milk protein and lactose intolerance are increasing day by day. Besides this, veganism (people strictly denies the consumption of animal products like milk, cheese, curd, yogurt, honey etc.) is becoming increasingly popular, so, the demand for lactose and cholesterol free, less in calories and cost effective beverage is increasing at a rapid pace. However in the past few years, food consumers have inclined towards plant-based diet which consists of components like cereal, legumes, seeds, nuts, fruits and vegetables because of factors like aversion to animal cruelty, wish for healthy lifestyle and environmental awareness. Such functional foods will be a boon for consumers with cowsmilk allergy, lactose intolerance, hypercholesterolemia and vegans etc. who will prefer the solid intakes and the beverages as well. This in turn demands for non-dairy based probiotic foods prepared from milk extracted from sources like coconut, cereals and legumes. Also, research shows that there is not much difference between cows milk and the milk obtained from plant legumes except the fat and calcium content and hence is considered a potent source of milk alternative which is not dairy base yet as nutritional as cows milk.

Cereals, as staple foods are consumed on a daily basis all over the world. They have complex nutrient composition and the daily consumption of cereals in India ranges from 60-80% of the daily energy requirement. Cereals are considered healthy non-dairy carriers to prepare probiotic foods as they can overcome the disadvantages of fermented dairy products like high cholesterol, calories and cost. Cereals are consumed as such and after processing in different forms like puffed wheat, rice flakes, malted beverages and many other form. Cereals along with pulses can be consumed in fermented form as *dosa, idli, dhokla* etc. Cereal grains like maize, sorghum, millet, oats, barley, wheat and rye are being used for this purpose. Intake of fermented cereals increases the availability of dietary fiber and non-digestible carbohydrates like oligosaccharides which acts as a prebiotic to stimulate the growth of probiotic LAB. Fermentation of cereals by *Lactobacillus* cultures is an oldest processing method used for the production of beverages, gruels and porridges in the countries of Asia and Africa. The consumption of whole grains increases the intake of fiber which binds the cholesterol and reduces the risk of cardiovascular diseases, obesity, certain type of cancers and type II diabetes mellitus.

ROLE OF SYNBIOTICS IN DISEASE MANAGEMENT

Synbiotics along with other natural foods are now considered essential resources to help sustain good health for humans and animals, for disease prevention and/or as alternatives to mitigate disease-related risks. Studies performed on the human gut and animal gut and immunology microbiota relationship have highlighted the role that synbiotics play in mammalian health. Synbiotics affect the microbial ecology of humans and animals' intestines, and play a role in reducing some diseases. They can be the safest and most efficient way to combat colonisation issues especially bacterial pathogens and infection with enteric pathogens. Functional prebiotic-like foods or natural antimicrobial supplements as alternatives and bioactive metabolite overexpression in probiotics are essential for improving synbiotic efficacy. Synbiotics can be effectively used as an immunity booster and in the management of obesity, Irritable Bowel Syndrome (IBS), Chronic Obstructive Pulmonary Diseases (COPD), type II diabetes mellitus etc.

Synbiotics for Chronic Bronchitis or Chronic Obstructive Pulmonary Disease

The concurrence of Chronic lung diseases, such as asthma and Chronic Obstructive Pulmonary Disease (COPD), with chronic gastrointestinal tract diseases, such as inflammatory bowel disease (IBD) or irritable bowel syndrome are often seen. These disease interrelationships suggest that there is an important bi-directional communication between the lung and the gut, known as the gut-lung axis, which may be influenced in part by communities of micro biota. The human micro biome is believed to contribute to homeostasis and disease, especially in the gut. Moreover, researches have shown that the gut micro biota vary with smoking status. Recently, a growing body of evidence has demonstrated that gut micro biota are closely related to respiratory health and disease, playing a vital role in the development of COPD, asthma, lung cancer and respiratory infections.

Synbiotics for Irritable Bowel Syndrome (IBS)

Probiotics have shown efficacy in the treatment and prevention of various medical conditions, especially those involving the gastrointestinal tract. Evidence supporting their position in certain situations is frequently in question. Probiotics demonstrate many ways of action: antagonism to pathogenic bacteria by production of products that inhibit their growth, such as bacteriocins, organic acids and hydrogen peroxide; or competing for locations adhering to the mucous membranes of the intestines; or competition for nutrients.

Alteration in the gut micro biota can cause, or aggravate, inflammatory bowel diseases. In patients with an inflammatory bowel disease, including infants, it is possible to play the therapeutic role of probiotics and prebiotics based on many animal trials and pilot human studies. Synbiotic treatment has been more widely employed in the treatment and care of gastro-intestinal disorders. It decreases IBD effects, boosts bacterial and viral immune systemic infection and removes diarrhoea triggered by antibiotics. In IBS patients it has been established that *haemophilusparainfluenzae* is more prevalent. Latest studies of micro biota have shown that adult bacterial intestinal dysbiosis can be decreased by the consumption of synbiotics.

Synbiotics as Potential Antioxidants

Probiotics can minimise the occurrence and length of diarrhoea, facilitate cell and mood tolerance, avoidance and adverse metabolism, like colon ammonium or pro cancerogenic enzymes. Furthermore, in recent years, several research have centred on the impact of intestinal micro biota on the health of a human. Metabolism by modulating intestinal microorganisms such as obesity and diabetes is classified as probiotics that could colonise the intestinal tract. The lactic acid (LAB) strains are the key players of the probiotic food and pharmaceutical industry. LABs have been found to promote ulcerative colitis (UC) prevention and repair. *Bifidobacteria* are a widely used probiotic bacterium. It will encourage tumour tolerance and mitigate women's irritable bowel syndrome. Due to their durability as sporal types of bacteria and their capacity to develop a number of enzymes including protease, amylase and lipase, species are favoured in the feed industry. In recent decades, numerous reports have shown the antioxidant ability of probiotics in addition to the favourable results.

Probiotics may generate different antioxidant metabolites such as butyrate, glutathione and folate. Folate is a vitamin used in a number of biochemical processes and takes place in a single carbon unit of donor molecules. Folate availability affects DNA replication, repair and methylation efficiency.

Synbiotics for boosting immunity

Chronic diseases associated with modern lifestyle habits are usually related to immune system malfunction. In this context, since diet is very well-known to modulate host resistance to infectious and inflammatory processes, the consumption of fibre and probiotics seems to be a promising nutritional tool for immune system modulation in different populations. Mechanisms may include modulation of the functional properties of the micro biota, epithelial cells, dendritic cells and immune cell types. The micro biome is an internal metropolis of trillions of microorganisms or microbes that live in our bodies, mostly in the intestines. These micro biome play a key role in immune function. The gut is a major site of immune activity and the production of antimicrobial proteins.

Dietary fibres can act as successful prebiotics by directly influencing the immune system and inducing dramatic adjustments in the intestinal microbial makeup, which can boost enteric inflamed-ness and systemic immune responses. The anti-inflammatory properties of fibre can be inducted by Short Chain Fatty Acids (SCFAs). SCFAs have been recognised as beneficial for bowel wellbeing for many decades. Prebiotics have been extensively reported to affect the composition of the gut micro biota, stimulating directly or indirectly putative beneficial gut commensals other than lactic acid bacteria. Age-related changes in gut physiology, micro biota and mucosal immune response are well established. Moreover, exposure to different challenges during life such as early encounter of environmental insults in the new-born, infant formula feeding, antibiotic treatment, gastrointestinal diseases and stress, also interferes with the normal development and balance of the healthy gut micro biota.

Synbiotics for Obesity

The importance of lactobacilli supplementation for adiposity management is advisable. The administration of various strains of Lactobacilli minimises the fat mass and the risk of type 2 diabetes mellitus and insulin resistance in individuals with obesity. Prebiotics which are the dietary fibres, helps in adding bulk to the food, gives satiety, binds the cholesterol, relieves constipation and thus, helps in managing the body weight.

Synbiotics and Diabetes

Synbiotics contribute to the specific improvements in gut micro biota, its composition and action and thus, helps in the management of diabetes. The prebiotics show selective stimulation of *bifidobacterial* and *lactobacillic* development contributing to major changes in intestinal micro biota composition.

Even after significant efforts to develop therapeutic solutions to metabolic issues and inflammatory disorders, these conditions are asking for urgent resolutions. It has been shown that many probiotic strains demonstrate health-improving factors leading to substantial changes within these conditions, but more reliable solutions remain paramount. A complex but positive gut ecosystem to human physiology through metabolic, and immuno-modulatory roles supports the concept of beneficial/probiotic bacteria, hence its modulation helps maintaining good health and lowers the risk of disease.

ROLE OF SYNBIOTICS IN RELIEVING THE SYMPTOMS OF COVID

The coronavirus disease-19 (COVID-19) is caused by SARS-CoV-2. It has massive global impact both on economy and human health. The most common symptoms of the disease are dry cough, fever, fatigue, myalgia, and dyspnea. It is also characterised by headache, sore throat, rhinorrhoea, and gastrointestinal disorders. Pneumonia appears to be the most common and severe manifestation of the infection. The infection is fatal also and it has been observed that some of the people died of cardiac arrest as its post impact. Currently, there is a vaccine for COVID-19 but it is still under study as people responded allergic reactions to it.

Further, the development of new antiviral which has positive impact requires a considerable length of time and effort for drug design and validation. Therefore, it is better to use natural compounds that can provide alternatives and can support therapy against COVID-19. The combination of probiotics and prebiotics i.e., synbiotics also play a unique role to modulate the gut microbe and assert gut homeostasis and production of interferon as an antiviral mechanism.

Administration of a balanced diet with good nutritional food habits can modulate the microbial community in the intestine. The synbiotic is safe and helpful in maintaining the gut micro biota, thus helpful in fighting with COVID-19 infection and relieving its symptoms. Probiotics are also responsible for reducing the risk of ventilator-associated pneumonia; other respiratory infection like chronic obstructive pulmonary diseases (COPD) etc.

The consumption of probiotics diminishes the danger of the basic cold and lessens the duration of the manifestations of respiratory tract infections. Probiotics, besides being beneficial bacteria, also possess antiviral activity and act as natural immune enhancers. Probiotics and their metabolites may also indirectly interfere with the virus by altering the state of cells, stimulating innate and/or adaptive immunity. They exert antiviral activity by-

(1) direct probiotic–virus interaction

(2) production of antiviral.

In a conclusion, globalisation, industrialisation and privatisation of jobs have adversely affected our life. We are now-a-days consuming fruits and vegetables loaded with fertilisers and pesticides, ready to eat or ready to cook foods are also full of food additives and preservatives. The air which we are breathing in is full of contaminants like heavy metals. So, the overall health of an individual is badly affected. COVID-19 pandemic has also contributed to the existing health conditions of people and has unfavourably affected it. The virus is transmitted through droplets i.e., when an infected person coughs or sneezes and also through the contact of surfaces containing the droplets that contain virus followed by touching nose, eyes, and mouth. The way virus is transmitted has led it spread globally. The spread of coronavirus can be prevented by boosting immunity by the consumption of antioxidant rich foods. These antioxidant rich foods can scavenge the free radicals produced in our body. Synbiotics, though are not a rich source of antioxidants but are a great choice for building immunity as they have both the live microorganisms as probiotics and the food for probiotics as prebiotics. So, when the gut health is improved, immunity is automatically built up. Regular consumption of synbiotic beverages can help in fighting COVID-19 infection by relieving its symptoms.

References

- Almeida, D., Machado, D., Andrade, J. C., Mendo, S., Gomes, A. M., & Freitas, A. C. (2020). Evolving trends in next-generation probiotics: a 5W1H perspective. *Critical Reviews in Food Science and Nutrition, 60*(11), 1783–1796. https://doi.org/10.1080/10408398.2019.1599812.

- Blandino, A., Al-Aseeri, M. E., Pandiella, S. S., Cantero, D. & Webb, C. (2003). Cereal-based fermented foods and beverages. *Food Res Int., 36*, 527–543. doi: 10.1016/S0963-9969(03)00009-7
- Budden, K. F., Gellatly, S. L. & Wood, D. L. (2017). Emerging pathogenic links between microbiota and the gut-lung axis. *Nat Rev Microbiol, 15,* 55–63.
- Bustamante, M., Oomah, B. D., Oliveira, W. P., Burgos-Díaz, C., Rubilar, M., & Shene, C. (2020). Probiotics and prebiotics potential for the care of skin, female urogenital tract, and respiratory tract. *Folia Microbiologica, 65*(2), 245–264. https://doi.org/10.1007/s12223-019-00759-3.
- Caballero, S. & Pamer, E. G. (2015). Microbiota-mediated inflammation and antimicrobial defense in the intestine. *Annual review of immunology, 21*(33), 227-256.
- Charalampopoulos, D., Wang, R., Pandiella, S. S. & Webb, C. (2002). Application of cereals and cereal components in functional foods: a review. *Int J Food Microbiol, 79,* 131–141. doi: 10.1016/S0168-1605(02)00187-3.
- Clemens, R. & Pressman, P. (2006). Heyday in grain land. *Food Technol., 60*(11), 18.
- Delzenne, N. M., Neyrinck, A. M., Bäckhed, F., & Cani, P. D. (2011). Targeting gut microbiota in obesity: effects of prebiotics and probiotics. *Nature Reviews Endocrinology, 7*(11), 639.
- Díaz, L. & Fernández-Ruiz, V. (2020). An international regulatory review of food health-related claims in functional food products labeling. *Elsevier*. https://www.sciencedirect.com/science/article/pii/S1756464620301201
- Dumas, A., Bernard, L., & Poquet, Y. (2018). The role of the lung microbiota and the gut-lung axis in respiratory infectious diseases. *Cell Microbiol, 20*, 1–9.
- Guillin, O.M., Vindry, C., Ohlmann, T. & Chavatte, L. (2019). Selenium, selenoproteins and viral infection. *Nutrients, 11*(9), 2101.
- Homayouni-rad, A., Torab, R., Ghalibaf, M., Norouzi, S. & Mehrabany, E. V. (2020). Evaluating the Role of Postbiotics as a New Generation of Probiotics in Health and Diseases. *Jarums.Arums.Ac.Ir., 30*(4), 430-435 http://jarums.arums.ac.ir/article-1-1766-en.pdf
- Keely, S., Talley, N. J. & Hansbro, P. M. (2012). Pulmonary-intestinal cross-talk in mucosal inflammatory disease. *Mucosal Immunol, 5,* 7–18.
- Lakshmi, B., Viswanath, B., Sai Gopal, D. V. R. (2013). Probiotics as antiviral agents in shrimp aquaculture. *J Pathogens, 21,* 1–13. https://doi.org/10.1155/2013/424123.
- Li, X. V., Leonardi, I. & Iliev, I. D. (2019). Gut microbiota in immunity and inflammatory disease. *Immunity, 50*(6), 1365-79.
- Malik, J. K., Ahmad, A. H., Kalpana, S., Prakash, A., & Gupta, R. C. (2016). Synbiotics: Safety and Toxicity Considerations. *Nutraceuticals: Efficacy, Safety and Toxicity*, 811–822. Elsevier Inc.https://doi.org/10.1016/B978-0-12-802147-7.00057-7
- Manigandan, T., Mangaiyarkarasi, S. P., Hemalatha, R., Hemalatha, V. T., & Murali, N. P. (2015). Probiotics, Prebiotics and Synbiotics– A Review.

Biomedical and Pharmacology Journal, *5*(2), 295–304. https://biomedpharmajournal.org/vol5no2/probiotics-prebiotics-and-synbiotics-a-review/

- Markowiak, P., & Z. lizewska, K. (2017). Effects of probiotics, prebiotics, and synbiotics on human health. *Nutrients*, *9*(9), 432-435. https://doi.org/10.3390/nu9091021.
- Merga, B., & Haji, J. (2019). Economic importance of Chickpea: Production, value, and world trade. *Cogent Food & Agriculture*, *5*(1). https://doi.org/10.1080/23311932.2019.1615718.
- Molendijk, I., Van der Marel, S. & Maljaars, P. W. (2019). Towards a Food Pharmacy: Immunologic Modulation through Diet. *Nutrients, 11*(6), 1239.
- Mortaz, E., Adcock, L. M., Folkerts, G., Barnes, P. J., Vos, A. P. & Garssen, J. (2013). Probiotics in the management of lung diseases. *MediatInflamm, 13,* 1–10. https://doi.org/10.1155/2013/751068.
- Pandey, K. R., Naik, S. R., & Vakil, B. V. (2015). Probiotics, prebiotics and synbiotics- a review. *Journal of Food Science and Technology, 52*(12), 7577–7587. https://doi.org/10.1007/s13197-015-1921-1.
- Prado, F. C., Parada, J. L., Pandey, A. & Soccol, C. R. (2008). Trends in non-dairy probiotic beverages. *Food Res Int., 41,* 111–123. doi: 10.1016/j.foodres.2007.10.010.
- Roobab, U., Batool, Z., Manzoor, M. F., Shabbir, M. A., Khan, M. R., & Aadil, R. M. (2020). Sources, formulations, advanced delivery and health benefits of probiotics. *Current Opinion in Food Science, 32,* 17–28. https://doi.org/10.1016/j.cofs.2020.01.003.
- Rutten, E. P. A., Lenaerts, K. & Buurman, W. A. (2014). Disturbed intestinal integrity in patients with COPD: effects of activities of daily living. *Chest, 145,* 245–52.
- Sankara, R. D. S. & Deosthale, Y. G. (1983). Mineral composition, ionizable iron and soluble zinc in malted grains of pearl millet and ragi. *Food Chem., 11,* 217–223. doi: 10.1016/0308-8146(83)90104-8.
- Sethi, S., Tyagi, S. K., & Anurag, R. K. (2016). Plant-based milk alternatives an emerging segment of functional beverages: a review. *Journal of Food Science and Technology, 53*(9), 3408–3423. https://doi.org/10.1007/s13197-016-2328-3.
- Wang, Y., Li, X., Ge, T., Xiao, Y., Liao, Y., Cui, Y., Zhang, Y., Ho, W., Yu, G. & Zhang, T. (2016). Probiotics for prevention and treatment of respiratory tract infections in children: A systematic review and meta-analysis of randomized controlled trials.*Medicine, 95,* e4509. https://doi.org/10.1097/MD.0000000000004509.
- Wessels, I., Maywald, M. & Rink, L. (2017). Zinc as a gatekeeper of immune function. *Nutrients, 9*(12), 1286.
- Williams, N. (2010). Probiotics. *Academic.Oup.Com.* https://academic.oup.com/ajhp/article-abstract/67/6/449/5130018.
- Wilson, B., & Whelan, K. (2017). Prebiotic inulin-type fructans and galacto-oligosaccharides: definition, specificity, function, and application in gastrointestinal disorders. *Journal of Gastroenterology and Hepatology,* 32, 64–68. https://doi.org/10.1111/jgh.13700.

8

Nutraceuticals and Functional Foods: Way for Healthy Life during and Post Covid-19

Dr Priyanka

Nutraceuticals and Functional foods are foods that offer health benefits beyond their nutritional value. The importance of nutraceuticals and functional foods products has been well recognised in connection with health promotion, disease risk reduction and immunity booster. Functional foods and nutraceuticals contain immune-boosting elements such as polyphenols, terpenoids, flavonoids, alkaloids, sterols, pigments, unsaturated fatty-acids, micronutrient vitamins and minerals, including vitamin A, B6, B12, C, D, E, and folate, and trace elements, including zinc, iron, selenium, magnesium, and copper. Foods with antiviral properties include fruits, vegetables, fermented foods and probiotics, olive oil, fish, nuts and seeds, herbs, roots etc. Nutraceuticals and Functional foods optimise the immune system capacity to prevent and control pathogenic viral infections. As we know COVID-19 pandemic is a serious *global* health threat, caused by a novel corona virus now called severe acute respiratory syndrome corona virus 2 (SARS-CoV-2; formerly called 2019-nCoV). In response to the Covid-19 pandemic, consumers are increasingly reaching for products that offer immunity boosting benefits as a preventative measure. The functional foods industry is seeing a rise in products that contain immune-boosting natural ingredients, such as turmeric, ginger and apple cider vinegar, as well as vitamins, minerals, prebiotics and probiotics.

A *nutraceutical* is defined as a food, food ingredients, and dietary *supplements* that provide health or medical benefits, or any product that is derived from food sources that offer extra health benefits in addition to the nutritional value of the food. They are the bioactive compounds found in fortified food, dietary supplements or herbal products. People are becoming more conscious of what they eat, as it becomes clear that poor nutritional habits can cause some of the serious diseases and health conditions out there. In India, nutraceuticals have been defined under Clause 22 of the Food Safety and Standards Act (FSSA), 2006. The term "nutraceutical" combines two words – "nutrient" (a nourishing food component) and "pharmaceutical" (a medical drug). The name was coined in 1989 by Stephen DeFelice, founder and chairman of the Foundation for Innovation in Medicine, an American organisation located in Cranford, New Jersey. Nutraceuticals play an important role in the therapeutic developments. A nutraceutical can be a nutrient-rich food, medicinally active food.

Nutraceuticals include **nutrients** such as minerals, vitamins, dietary fibres, hydrolyzed proteins, fortified foods, prebiotics, probiotics, polyunsaturated fatty acids, antioxidants, **dietary supplement** (a product that contains nutrients derived from food products, and is often concentrated in liquid, capsule, powder or pill form. Although dietary supplements are regulated by the FDA as foods, their regulation differs from drugs and other foods). **Herbs** are plants with fragrant or aromatic properties. *Herbs* can be used to flavour food, included in fragrances, and even a part of natural medicines. India has a very long history of safely using many *herbs.* The traditional medical properties seek to normalise body functions with varied techniques including food and activity. Herbs which are commonly used ajwain, ashwagandha, cardamom, cumin, licorice, manjistha, neem, shatavari, turmeric, haritaki, aleovera, etc.

Functional foods are foods that offer health benefits beyond their nutritional value. It contains bioactive compounds naturally. Significantly, these foods can provide health benefits beyond the traditional nutritional value of the food. Here, the traditional nutrients refer to the regular vitamins and minerals found in that particular food. Functional foods can be considered to be those whole, fortified, enriched or enhanced foods that provide health benefits beyond the provision of essential nutrients (e.g., vitamins and minerals). That foods might provide therapeutic benefits.

Functional foods	***Bioactive components***
Soy	Protein
Whole oat products	β-Glucan
Cranberry juice	Proanthocyanidins
Fatty fish	(n-3) Fatty acids
Garlic	Organosulfur compounds
Green tea	Catechins
Spinach, kale, collard greens	Lutein/zeaxanthin
Tomatoes and processed tomato products	Lycopene

Bioactive compounds have actions in the body that may promote good health. Several functional foods interact with the epigenetic regulation of viral infection and mechanisms of senescence. Immunity plays an important role in covid-19. A type of chemical found in small amounts in plants and certain foods (such as fruits, vegetables, nuts, oils, and whole grains). Bioactive compounds have actions in the body that may promote good health. They are being studied in the prevention of cancer, heart disease, and other diseases. Examples of bioactive compounds include lycopene, resveratrol, lignan, tannins, and indoles.

The immune system protects against viruses and diseases and produces antibodies to kill pathogens. A study also found that people who have recovered from Covid-19 have powerful and protective killer immune cells even when antibodies are not detectable. Because there is no registered medicine or vaccine against COVID-19, the immune system is the best defense because it supports the body's natural ability to defend against pathogens (e.g., viruses, bacteria, fungi, protozoan, and worms) and resists infections. After being affected by virus immune responses to mediate antibody. The B cells are assisted by T cells to differentiate into plasma cells, which then produce antibodies specific to a viral antigen. A neutralising nature antibody is efficient in fully blocking the virus from entering into host cells to limit the infection and plays a very intense protective role at the later stage of infection and prevents relapse of infection.

As above described the responsibility of immune system the need is quick boost to the immunity system to keep it fighting fit.*Nutraceuticals*, *Functional foods*, and Dietary *supplements* (NFD) such as:Copper, Folate, Iron, Selenium, Zinc, probiotics, selenium and dietary antioxidants (vitamins A, E and C) oil capsules, herb extracts, glucosamine and chondroitin sulfate pills, lutein-containing multivitamin tablets etc., *important* in maintaining and/or improving *immune function.*

Covid -19 makes people more conscious about their health, immunity, and healthy lifestyle. While no foods or dietary supplements can prevent COVID-19 infection, but by maintaining a healthy diet we can keep our immune system strong for fighting the disease. The tenet, "Let food be thy medicine and medicine be thy food" was embraced 2500 years ago by Hippocrates, the father of medicine. Nutraceuticals and functional foods have plenty of medical properties which help to makes body healthy. Every day, eat a combination of different foods including whole grains such as wheat, maize and rice, legumes like lentils and beans, fruits and vegetables and some foods from animal sources (e.g. meat, fish, eggs and milk). Eat fresh fruit and vegetables.Using a variety of *herbs* in your diet *will* not only please your taste buds, it will help to provide natural medicine and enhance immunity.*Kitchen* garden is the treading way to use and harvest fresh *herbs*, Tulsi, Mentha, Coriander and Curry leaves are the most popular *kitchen herbs* in India.

Most of the organisations and societies recommended avoiding the intake of salt, fat, and sugar and encouraged reductions in sugary drinks, other sugar-rich products, meat portions, and other foods of animal origin to lower the intake of saturated fat. In addition, it was suggested that low-fat dairy foods and healthy fats (e.g., olive oil and fish oil) be included in the diet and recommended sauces, spices, and herbs as salt substitutes.

It has described a definitive role of fat in immunity. Saturated fatty acids act on Toll-like receptor 4, a sensor that binds bacterial lipopolysaccharide and thus acts in the innate immune response. As a result, a high intake of saturated fatty acids favours low-grade inflammation. On the other hand, monounsaturated and polyunsaturated fatty acids are known for their favourable immune-modulatory action. Omega-3 polyunsaturated fatty acids present in seafood, algal oil, marine fish, and flaxseed support the immune system by activating cells from both the innate and the adaptive immune systems, while omega-9 monounsaturated fatty acids found in olive, sunflower, and safflower oils and nuts have antioxidant, antimicrobial, and antiviral effects. For adult males and nonpregnant/nonlactating adult females, the recommended dosage of omega-3 polyunsaturated fatty acids (eicosapentaenoic acid plus docosahexaenoic acid) is 250 mg/d. This recommendation can be met by consuming at least 2 portions (90 g each) of fatty marine fish, such as mackerel, salmon, sardine, herring, and smelt, per week.

In kitchen hygiene is also important factor for healthy living so keep clean; separate raw and cooked food; cook thoroughly; keep food at safe temperatures; use safe water and sanitize raw materials to prevent the Covid-19 viral infection, any other viral, bacterial, and food-borne illnesses. Drink enough water and stay hydrated.Wear a face mask or cloth cover while in public. Hands should be sanitized every 20-30 minutes. Physical activity and exercise should include in daily routine. Aim to get some type of exercise most days such as run, walk, cycling or swim outdoors, benefits both physically and psychologically. Not only will you get the benefits of exercise, spending time in nature has been shown to have a positive impact on mood.

Living a *healthy* lifestyle is one of the most important things you could do for yourself. A *healthy* lifestyle focuses on physical and mental well-being. Include healthy food which should be rich in a variety of functional foods, nutraceuticals including various nutrients. These foods not only supply your body with the vitamins and minerals it needs but also support overall health.

This review summarises recent scientific literature on an optimal diet, vitamin and mineral supplementation, and good hygiene practices for food preparation during the COVID-19 pandemic. The findings can be used to help dietitians and healthcare professionals better address dietary recommendations during the COVID-19 pandemic. Guidance related to the safe handling of food, from production to consumption, is critical to reduce the risk of viral dissemination. The general recommendation is to consume a diet based predominantly on fresh foods such as fruits, vegetables, whole grains, low-fat dairy sources, and healthy fats (olive oil and fish oil) and to limit intakes of sugary drinks and processed foods high in calories and salt. Dietary supplements (i.e., vitamins C and D, zinc, and selenium) should be administered to individuals with, or at risk of, respiratory viral infections or in whom deficiency is detected. Breast milk is the safest and healthiest food for infants, and breastfeeding should be encouraged, even in women diagnosed with COVID-19.

References

1. Zhao, J. Bentham Science Publishers; 2007. Nutraceuticals, Nutritional Therapy, Phytonutrients, and Phytotherapy for Improvement of Human Health: A Perspective on Plant Biotechnology Application.
2. Kalra, EK. Nutraceutical – Definition and introduction. AAPS Pharm Sci. 2003; 5: E25.
3. Chauhan, B, Kumar, G, Kalam, N, Ansari, SH. Current concepts and prospects of herbal nutraceutical: A review. J Adv Pharm Technol Res. 2013; 4: 4–8.
4. Zeisel, SH. Regulation of "nutraceuticals" Science. 1999; 285: 1853–5.
5. Hardy, G. Nutraceuticals and functional foods: Introduction and meaning. Nutrition. 2000; 16: 688–9.
6. Baradaran, A, Madihi, Y, Merrikhi A, Rafieian-Kopaei, M, Nasri, H. Serum lipoprotein (a) in diabetic patients with various renal function not yet on dialysis. Pak J Med Sci. 2013; 29(Suppl): 354–7.
7. Nasri, H. Impact of diabetes mellitus on parathyroid hormone in hemodialysis patients. J Parathyr Dis. 2013; 1: 9–11.
8. Gombart, AF, Pierre, A, Maggini, S. A review of micronutrients and the immune system—working in harmony to reduce the risk of infection. Nutrients. 2020; 12: 236.
9. Institute of Medicine, Panel on Dietary Reference Intakes for Electrolytes and Water. *Dietary Reference Intakes for Water, Potassium, Sodium, Chloride, and Sulfate.*

10. Popkin, BM, D'Anci, KE, Rosenberg, IH. Water, hydration, and health. Nutr Rev. 2010; 68: 439–458.
11. Brower, V. Nutraceuticals: Poised for a healthy slice of the healthcare market? Nat Biotechnol, 1998; 16: 728-31.
12. Trottier G, Boström PJ, Lawrentschuk, N, Fleshner, NE. Nutraceuticals and prostate cancer prevention: A current review. Nat Rev Urol 2010; 7: 21-30.
13. Kalra, EK. Nutraceutical - Definition and introduction. AAPS PharmSci 2003; 5: E25.
14. Zeisel, SH. Regulation of "Nutraceuticals". Science 1999; 285: 1853-5.
15. Dillard, CJ, German, JB. Phytochemicals: Nutraceuticals and human health. J Sci Food Agric 2000; 80: 1744-56.

9

Immunity Learning Policy for School Going Children: Need and Awareness

Dr Sukanya Chakravorty

The school environment is a natural entry point for reaching children and adolescents with health education, health promotion and health services. Schools present the ideal ecosystem for students to imbibe from peers and learn from role models, such as teachers and head of school. Students can be effective advocates for creating a healthy school and can become change agents for the community health initiatives. Health and Education are strongly connected. Healthy children achieve better results at school, which in turn are associated with improved health later in life. Setting up positive and healthy school environment, then, plays an important role in improving the health, well-being, overall academic achievement.

Healthy children are the foundation for a healthy nation and nation's future depends on the status of the children. Leaders around the world have acknowledged schools as an important setting where children develop behaviour skills for physical, emotional and social well-being. Other than the family, no social institution has greater influence on the lives of children than schools. Every day millions of children in the country go to school and spend a considerable amount of time interacting with their peers and teachers gaining knowledge, building attitudes and skills, and developing behaviours. Behavioural patterns that develop during childhood and adolescence are retained for life.

Health and Education are strongly interconnected. While healthy individuals are more likely to have better outcomes, right education can improve the health status of a household but in context of India, we need to do more to create awareness amongst school going children about immunity and health. During this pandemic time, this is the need indeed to enrich all school going children with the root health and immune policy. Recently Indian government released National Education Programme 2020 (NEP) which proposes to bring a paradigm shift in Indian education. In doing so, it recognizes the need for nourishment and good health to aid optimal learning, and proposes certain health-related interventions.

The following are the key approaches and interventions on health proposed in the NEP.

Holistic education with sports-integration

Multidisciplinary and holistic education is part of the key principles of the NEP. Along with subjects like social sciences, the curriculum must contain courses that make education well-rounded, useful and fulfill games, sports and fitness. At the school level, the NEP proposes sports-integration, or utilising physical activities in pedagogical practice students' cognitive abilities, while promoting their physical and psychological well-being. Sports help students achieve fitness levels envisaged in the Fit India movement, and adopt fitness for lifelong to develop their skills like collaboration, self-initiative, teamwork and responsibility.

The NEP also proposes other ways to increase school students' exposure to sports and other activities. It offers flexibility and choice of subjects, allowing students to choose physical education as part of the curriculum proposes 'bagless' days to allow students to engage in local vocational and other activities, such as sport. The NEP further encourages formation of clubs, including for sports, yoga, and health and well- being, at the levels of schools, school complexes, districts and beyond.

Expansion of food programme

India's mid-day meal programme exemplifies the convergence of education with a food and nutrition pro. Currently, mid-day meals are provided to children in Classes 1 to 8, studying primarily in government and aided schools. The NEP proposes provision for early child care education.

Further, NEP proposes provision of breakfast for school children in addition to mid-day meals, so that the child portrays increased productivity during morning hours after a healthy breakfast, especially for the study of subjects. Where serving cooked meals is not feasible, breakfast may include simple-yet-nutritious foods groundnuts/chana with jaggery and/ or fruits.

Health education

Noting the importance of health education in schools, the NEP includes health and nutrition, physical education wellness, sports, sanitation and hygiene as some of the key subjects, skills and capacities that must be liked by everyone. Accordingly, the NEP proposes the inclusion of training in health, including preventive health, good nutrition, personal and public hygiene, disaster response and first-aid, and detrimental effects of other drugs, as part of the school curriculum. The increasing prevalence of non-communicable diseases and intake of poor diets, may lead to behaviour change towards healthier habits. However, the NEP does not provide any roadmap or framework for inclusion of health education in the curriculum, and much will depend upon implementation of the Policy.

Healthy learning environments

This includes regularity in schools, especially for 100% immunisation, and health monitoring through health cards. Children are vulnerable to wide spectrum of communicable and chronic disease conditions including nutritional deficiencies, substance abuse, mental health concerns, violence, injury and reproductive and sexual health problems. A number of these issues can be prevented through informed health choices. A focused and comprehensive intervention that targets risk factors and social determinants of health conditions as well as empowers children and adolescents to adopt healthy behaviours can play an important role in reducing the burden of these diseases. More children than ever are attending school, and for longer periods of their lives, therefore, schools can do more than perhaps any other single institution to improve the wellbeing and competence of children and adolescents. It is a well-known fact that establishing healthy behaviours during childhood is easier and more effective that trying to change unhealthy during adulthood. Therefore, schools play a critical role in helping students establish healthy behaviours for their lifetime. Thus, the Department of School Education, Ministry of Human Resource Development and Ministry of Health and Family Welfare are proposing a joint initiative to improve the health of school children under AYUSHMAN BHARAT. Two teachers in every school will be declared as "Health and Wellness Ambassadors" preferably one male and one female and who will transact weekly health promotion and disease prevention information in the form of interactive activities.

Addressing critical health challenges

Taking a forward-looking approach, the NEP highlights the need to develop an education system that address its key challenges, including in health. This will require high-quality studies in science, social science, humanities, interdisciplinary research, and other advancements in the education system. India should also cutting-edge areas, such as artificial intelligence, big data and genomic studies. These studies can have applications in critical areas, including health.

The NEP further notes the need to improve professional education in certain fields; including agriculture. An Agriculture education should be able to develop professionals who can address issues related to food and land productivity. Healthcare education should be re-envisioned to make the programme more focused on preventive healthcare and community medicine.

Although providing a healthy environment to a child can include other aspects, the NEP takes a step towards education and health to enable children to learn and grow as healthy individuals.

Because schools materially influence both health and education, they substantially determine the future well-being and economic productivity of populations. Recent research suggests that healthier children learn better and that more educated adults are healthier. School health is a cross-disciplinary field of study and a fundamental strategy that can be used to improve both health and education outcomes. Modern school health programmes include 10 interactive components: health education; physical education and physical activity; nutrition environment and services; health services; counselling, psychological, and social services; physical environment; social and emotional climate; family engagement; community involvement; and employee wellness. This review is written for both health and education audiences. It integrates recent research and developments in relationships among health, education, and economic outcomes; health and education systems; the school health programme, its components, and their effectiveness; cross-disciplinary collaboration; local, state, national, and international infrastructures and strategies; implementation science; and relevant academic research, training, and service.

Worldwide, about 1.3 billion young people are enrolled in primary and secondary schools across 241 countries. In the United States, about 130,000 public and private schools, in 13,000 school districts, employ 6 million teachers and students educate 55 million prekindergarten through grade 12 (PK–12) students every school day, usually for 13 of the most formative years of their lives. Among these students, 27% live in another-only household; 20% live in poverty; 13% receive special education services for disabilities; and 9% are non-English-speaking learners. In a given year, 13–20% of children experiences a mental disorder, including anxiety, depression, behavioral or conduct problems, attention-deficit/hyperactivity disorder, and autism spectrum disorders. These disorders appear to be increasing. In 2017, 40% of high school students had engaged in sexual intercourse, 39% texted or emailed while driving, 30% used alcohol, 23% had asthma, 20% used marijuana, 16% were overweight, 15% had obesity, 14% inappropriately used prescription pain medicine, 13% used an electronic vapour product, 9% smoked cigarettes, and 7% had attempted suicide. In 2015, among 71 nations, US students ranked twenty-third in reading, twenty-fifth in science, and thirty-ninth in mathematics.

A small set of common risk factors are responsible for most of the major causes; **unhealthy diet, physical inactivity** and **tobacco use**. Elimination of the modifiable risk factors would prevent 80% of premature heart disease, 80% of premature stroke, 80% of type 2 diabetes and 40% of cancer. Children are not immune to this burden. Overweight children and obesity and type 2 diabetes in children and adolescents are an increasing problem. Globally, nearly 22 million children under 5 years of age are overweight. Overweight and obese children are likely to stay obese in adulthood.

Need of training of children to build immune systems develop, ability to fight off germs will follow:

Building immunity

Children need exposure to microbes/germs – and the resulting illnesses – to develop strong immune systems. Basically, people have two-part immune systems.

1st-We're born with "**innate**" immunity that helps prevent infection. Skin is a part of it, helping to ward off invading organisms.

2nd- **"Adaptive"** or **"acquired"** immunity builds up over time as a child is exposed to more and more microbes. It's based completely on the pathogens we're exposed to. Each illness, and each vaccine, teaches the immune system how to fight off a new pathogen. With each new pathogen a child encounters, their immune system gets more "experienced."

Our immune systems need to be stronger to fight with all-time available viruses and bacteria.

Some ways to help kids' immune systems:

- **Make sure they get plenty of sleep.**

  The role of sleep in a child's immune system is huge. If your child's not getting enough sleep, they're going to be more susceptible to illness.

  Citing connections between sufficient sleep and disease prevention, the Centers for Disease Prevention and Control recommends 12 to 14 hours for 1- to 3-year-olds; 11 to 13hours for 3- to 5-year-olds; and 10 to 11 hours for children ages 5 to 10. Adolescents need more sleep than adults, the health experts says – 8.5 to 9.5 hours for 10- to 17-year-olds.

- **Give them a variety of healthy foods.**

  Experts advised lots of fruits and vegetables and grains and minimising foods containing simple sugars. It's old advice that's forgotten as families get busy and parents seek out easy – salty, sugary, fatty – offerings. As humans we want what we can quickly and easily get.

- **Strive for at least 60 minutes of exercise and yoga a day.**

  Kids need an hour of "rigorous" activity daily, something to get their heart rate up, whether it's soccer or going on a bike ride. With increased blood flow, they're increasing oxygen to the brain and other organs and over because it's been shown, over and over, to be the best way to prevent the spread of germs.

- **Sneeze wisely.**

  Teach children to do the "vampire cough" when they don't have a tissue on hand – sneezing or coughing into the inside of their elbow to minimize germs sent airborne.

- **Teach children to be germ-aware.**

  Encourage them to throw away their used tissues and avoid using other children's cups. Younger kids, especially, need help keeping their fingers away from their mouths and noses, those orifices are the germ playgrounds.

  With each passing year, more and more children are diagnosed with various health issues. From a lack of school health staff to severe allergies, check out 5 of the biggest health concerns that K-12 schools nationwide face.

No School Nurse

When a kid gets sick at school, generally they go to the school nurse. But, at many schools that don't employ a full-time registered nurse, that's not possible. Additionally, the question of who takes responsibility for student health records comes up. If there aren't any full-time nurses, does the burden then fall to a part-time health staff employee? How are all of the day-to-day administrative and clinical tasks communicated? All it would take is just one small misstep with a student's medication or an athlete's concussion rehab track for a substantial liability case. In situations like this, communication and coordination are critical to a successful school health department. Ideally, every school would have at least 1 full-time nurse, but since that is not an option, its crucial that schools house their student health information in one secure, centralised location, where all health staff, even rotating personnel, can access the information to coordinate better student care.

School Environment

Policy and Administrative Support

District policies and administrative guidelines reflect a commitment to maintaining an open and positive psychosocial climate and a healthy physical environment that are conducive to high student achievement and the long-term health of students and staff. Policies, rules and regulations are consistently enforced. The chief administrator, the school board and the school health coordinating council receive, at least annually, a report on the psychosocial climate of the school and a report on the physical environment, along with an action plan for continuous improvement of the school environment. Effort should be made to compare the progress in the psychosocial and physical health awareness with relevant educational goals. Policies that assure safe transport of students to and from school (e.g., bus, bicycle, walking) are enforced.

Psychosocial Environment

Administrative support for a healthy psychosocial environment is evidenced by district and campus policies and procedures. The school environment is friendly, nurturing, physically and emotionally safe and conducive to learning with high expectations for academic success.

School climate problems are addressed directly, in a timely manner and discussed openly within the limits of privacy. Effective instructional plans and techniques are used with all students to foster learning, self-worth and mental health. Students, families and staff work as a team in planning and implementing programmes and activities to affirm all cultural, linguistic and socioeconomic backgrounds. Students, families and staff are regarded as valuable and are involved in school governance. Students are empowered to take a leadership role in the development and implementation of programmes to promote a healthy school. Focus is placed on people's feelings and needs as well as tasks and duties.

Health Education

Policy and Administrative Support

District policies and administrative guidelines reflect a commitment to attain desired student outcomes essential to optimal physical and mental health. The chief administrator of the school board and the school health coordinating council receive, at least annually, reports on actions taken and results achieved related to desired student outcomes, along with the action plan for continuous improvement in health education. At the intermediate and secondary level, certified health education specialists with teacher certification teach the health courses. Coordination and team teaching with related professionals is encouraged. At the elementary level, teachers have professional preparation in elementary health education. Educators are given opportunities for effective professional training when implementing a new curriculum.

Goals and Objectives

District/school goals and objectives for health education are clear, based on assessed needs and stated in terms of student outcomes expected at each grade level and for each course.

References

1. Adapted from Consensus Statement on School Health. Canadian Association for School Health.
2. Adapted from the Report of the 1990 Joint Committee on Health Education Terminology. J Sch Health1991;61(6):251-254.
3. Comprehensive school health education. New Delhi, WHO Regional Office for South-East Asia, 1993.
4. Fruit and vegetables for health. Report of a joint FAO/WHO Workshop. Geneva, World Health Organization, 2004.
5. Global Strategy on Diet, Physical Activity and Health. Geneva, World Health Organization, 2004.

6. Global strategy on diet, physical activity and health: a framework to monitor and evaluate implementation. Geneva, World Health Organization, 2006.
7. Guidelines for Comprehensive School Health Programs - Schools & Health - NCBI Bookshelf Healthy nutrition: an essential element of a health-promoting school. Geneva, World Health Organization, 1998 (WHO Information Series on School Health, Document No. 4).
8. Integrated management of healthy settings at the district level. Geneva, World Health Organization, 2002.
9. National Committee for Health Education Credentialing, Inc; 1991.
10. Nutrition-friendly schools initiative, Part I: NFSI Framework. Geneva, World Health Organization, 2007.
11. Operational Guidelines on School Health Programme under Ayushman Bharat Health and Wellness Ambassadors partnering to build a stronger future, A Joint initiative of Ministry of Health & Family Welfare and Ministry of Human Resource & Development, April 2018
12. Outcomes of Quality Physical Education Programs. National Association for Sport and Physical Education: 1992.
13. Preventing chronic diseases, a vital investment. Geneva, World Health Organization, 2005.
14. Proctor, ST, Lordi, SL, Zaiger, DS. School Nursing Practice Roles and Standards. National Association of School Nurses, Inc., Scarborough, ME: 1993;18.
15. Programme for Nutrition and Food Security. Copenhagen, World Health Organization, WHO Regional Office for Europe, 2006.
16. Promoting physical activity in schools: an important element of a health-promoting school. Geneva, World Health Organization, 2006 (WHO Information Series on School Health, Document No. 12).
17. Responsibilities and competencies for entry-level health educators. Provider Designation Handbook. New York.
18. The status of school health. Geneva, World Health Organization, 1996.
19. These standards for school nursing practice are based upon Standards of Clinical Nursing Practice. Washington, DC: American Nurses' Publishing; 1991.
20. https://www.covid19.qld.gov.au
21. https://www.healthychildren.org/English/ages-stages/gradeschool/school/Pages/Health-Problems-at-School.aspx
22. https://medlineplus.gov/schoolhealth
23. https://www.ncbi.nlm.nih.gov

10

Phytochemicals and Nutraceuticals-Effective Agents against COVID-19

Dr Sangeeta

During this pandemic of COVID-19 when the data of all positive cases of corona has reached around millions and deaths rate is also very critical worldwide, excessive number of deaths occurred in America, which gives a critical graph of a developed country where medical facilities are on the top level of world but here they found to be helpless in this crisis. Even though now treatment or vaccine for this virus is available, the health scientists and doctors have advised to consume nutritious and immunity booster foods which can protect us from the virus infection and develop immunity to fight against the virus. Phytochemicals are non-nutritive bioactive secondary compounds abundantly found in fruits, grains, and vegetables. Consumption of phytochemicals may protect against chronic diseases like cardiovascular disease, neurodegenerative disease, and cancer, and also increases the immunity which fights with virus. Foods high in photochemical are also important for wellness. Phytochemical appear in all plants, therefore, a diet that includes a variety of grains, fruits, and vegetables will provide these healthy substances .Foods rich in phytochemical include apples, apricots, broccoli, Brussels sprouts, cabbage, carrots, cauliflower, garlic, legumes, onions, red peppers, soybeans, sweet potatoes, and tomatoes. Researches and evidences reveal that phytochemical foods are also known as super foods which are helpful in maintaining good health and boost immunity as well. Neutraceuticals and probiotics are also included in building up the best immunity.

Phytochemicals are non-nutritive plants chemical that have protective properties. More than thousand of phytochemicals are present in nature which are beneficial for the health. Plant produces theses chemicals that are very effective for us to protect ourselves from many diseases. Some known phytochemical are lycopene in tomatoes, flavonoids in fruits, and isoflavones in soya. These major phytochemicals are essential for sustaining good health and human life.

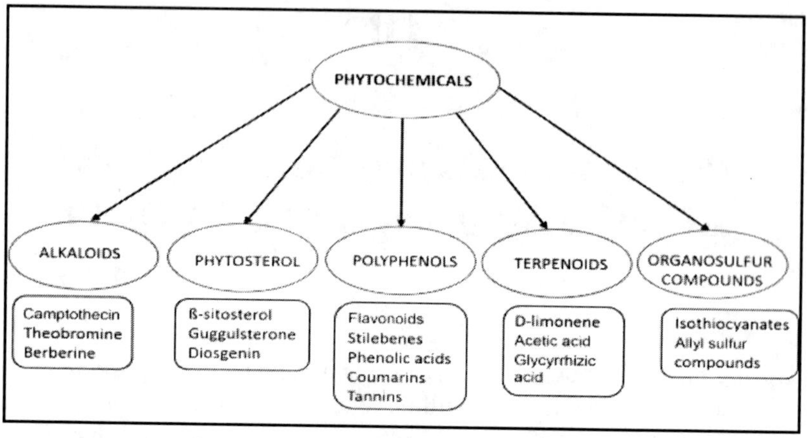

Fig. 1: Types of Phytochemical.

Color	Phytochemicals	Fruits and vegetables
Red	Lycopene	Tomatoes and tomato products such as juice, soups, and pasta sauces
Red-Purple	Anthocyanins and polyphenols	Grapes, blackberries, red wine, raspberries, blueberries
Orange	Alpha and beta-carotene	Carrots, mangos, pumpkin
Orange-Yellow	Beta-cryptoxanthin and flavonoids	Cantaloupe, peaches, tangerines, papaya, oranges
Yellow-Green	Lutein and zeaxanthin	Spinach, avocado, honeydew melon
Green	Glucosinolates and indoles	Broccoli, bok choi, kale
White-Green	Allyl sulfides	Leeks, garlic, onion, chives

Fig. 2: Phytochemical in various food products.

Neutraceutical arose first in the survey from U.K., Germany and France, where diet was rated higher by the consumers than exercise or hereditary factors to achieve a good health. Neutraceutical covers most of the therapeutic areas such as anti-arthritic, cold and cough, sleeping disorders, digestion and prevention of certain cancers, osteoporosis, blood pressure, cholesterol control, pain killers, depression and diabetes. Neutraceuticals are the supplement with nutrition and pharmaceutical, it could be defined as food which help in prevention of diseases and protect from many infectious diseases. COVID- 19 is mRNA virus which spreads through the human to human and air as well. Neutraceuticals include natural product, herbal and dietary supplement, these three segments are helpful in improving immunity and protecting form infections. This pandemic raised the importance of natural care for boosting immunity and fighting against the virus.

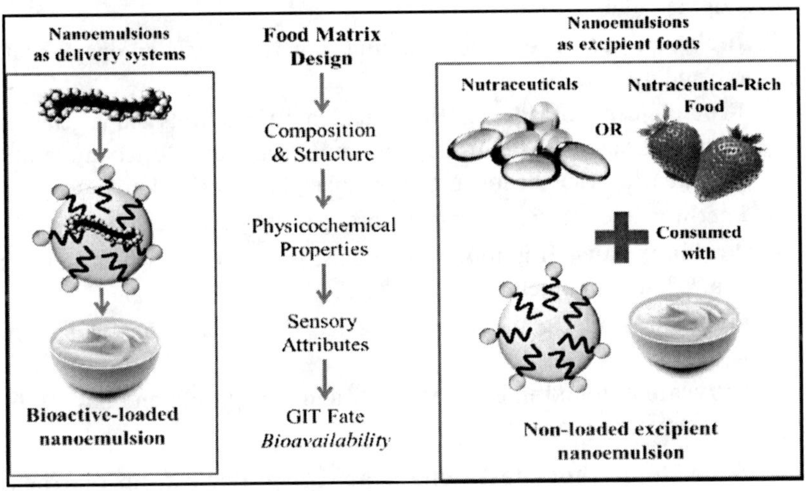

Image 1: Mechanisms of Neutraceutical.

A food or beverage product containing ingredients or structures that increases the bioavailability of drug or Neutraceutical that it is consume with.

Food sources used as Neutraceutical can be categorised as: Dietary fiber, Probiotics, Prebiotic, Polyunsaturated fatty acids, Antioxidants vitamins, Polyphones and spices. These all foods are also known as super food and help to boost immunity level. Prebiotic are a compound that induce the growth and activity of beneficial microorganisms in the gastrointestinal tract and helps to improve gut health and activity which are responsible for good immune system and health.

Prebiotics are specialised plant fibers found in many fruits and vegetables.It is complex carbohydrate, fiber and starch.They act as fertilisers and stimulate growth of good bacteria.

Prebiotic are types of dietary fiber that feed the friendly bacteria inside the gut. It helps the gut bacteria to produce nutrients for our colon cell and leads to a healthier digestive system, e.g. short chain fatty acid like: butyrate acetate and propionate, produce in gut friendly bacteria and plays a crucial role in health or immunity and reduces risk of inflammatory disease, type 2 diabetes, obesity, heart disease and other complications. About 95% of the short chain fatty acid in our body are: acetate (C2), propionate (C3) and butyrate (C4).

Following fibers are best for the production of short fatty chain fatty acids in the colon:

Inulin- present in sufficient amount in garlic, leeks, onions, wheat, rye and asparagus.

Fructoligoshacharides (FOS) –found in various fruits and vegetables including bananas, onions, garlic and asparagus, Resistant starch-grain, barley, rice, beans, green bananas, legumes and potatoes.

Pectin- apples, apricots, carrots, oranges etc.

Arabinoxylane- It is found in cereals, grains, e.g. - wheat bran. It has 70% fiber content.

Guar gum-Guar gum can be extracted from guar beans which are legumes.

Butyrate's- found in cheese, butter and cow's milk and have anti-inflammatory properties.

Benefits of short fatty chain acid – protects from diarrhea, inflammatory bowl disease (IBD). Short-chain fatty acids have been shown to protect against colon cancer in animal and lab studies. Short-chain fatty acid and diabetes positive effects in both animals and humans with type 2 diabetes. The same review also highlighted that there appears to be an imbalance in gut microorganism in people with diabetes.

Dietary fiber is the food material, more precisely the plant material that is not hydrolyzed by enzymes secreted by the digestive tract, but digested by microflora in the gut. Dietary fibers mostly include non-starch polysaccharides (NSP) such as celluloses, hemicelluloses, gums and pectin's, lignin, resistant dextrin and resistant starches. Foods rich in soluble fiber include fruits, oats, barley and beans. Chemically dietary fiber means carbohydrate polymers with a degree of polymerisation not lower than 3, which are neither digested nor absorbed in the small intestine. Based on their water solubility, dietary fibers may be divided into two forms:-

Insoluble dietary fiber (IDF), which includes celluloses, some hemi-celluloses and lignin's which is fermented to a limited extend in the colon.

Soluble dietary fiber (SDF), which includes β-glucans, pectin's, gums, mucilage and hemicelluloses that are fermented in the colon.

Table 1: The level of dietary fiber in certain foods has been illustrated

Product	*AOAC(g/100gm)*
Apples (with Skin)	2.0
Bananas	1.9
Carrots (Boiled)	3.1
Baked Beans	4.2
Cabbage	2.0
White Bread	2.0
Brown Bread	4.5
Whole meal Bread	7.4

Source: AOAC values *CRC Handbook of Dietary Fiber in Human Nutrition,* 2nd edition (1993).

Persons consuming generous amount of dietary fiber, compared to those who have minimal fiber intake, are having low risk of CHR (Liu *et al.,* 1999), stroke (Steffen *et al.,* 2003), hypertension (Whelton *et al.,* 2005), diabetes (Montonen *et al.,* 2003), obesity (Lairon *et al.,* 2005) and certain gastrointestinal disorders (Petruzziello *et al.,* 2006). Again, increase in the intake of high fiber food improves serum lipoprotein values (Brown *et al.,* 1999), lowers blood pressure level (Keenan *et al.,* 2002), improves blood glucose control for diabetes (Anderson *et al.,* 2004), aids weight loss (Birketvedt *et al.,* 2005) and promotes regularity (Cummings, 2001). Research reveals that certain soluble fibers enhance the immunity in humans (Watzl *et al.,* 2005). Some potential negative effects of dietary fiber include reduced absorption of vitamins, minerals, proteins and calories. It is recommended that dietary fiber intake for adults generally fall in the range of 20–35 g/day (Pilch, 1987). The recommended dietary fiber intake for children and adults are estimated to be 14 g/1,000 kCals (Anderson *et al.,* 2009). Several case histories have reported that consumption of excessive amounts of dietary fiber causes diarrhea (Saibil, 1989).

SARS-CoV-2 is mRNA virus with a genetic structure similar to that of SARS-CoV or MERS-CoV. The viral genome encodes a protease, which plays a crucial role in the production of viral proteins and controlling the activity of the replicase complex. This enzyme is necessary for virus replication and infection, making it a perfect target for designing antiviral therapies. Acute respiratory syndrome (SARS-CoV) coronavirus enzymes are one of the most promising targets for the discovery of anti-SARS drugs because of its key role in the life cycle of the virus. Natural inhibitors like betulinic acid, indigo, aloeemodine, luteolin, and quinomethyl triterpenoids, quercitin or gallates can be effective as antiviral preparations.

The SARS-CoV-2 genome is composed of approximately 30,000 nucleotides (Jin *et al.,* 2020) and codes, 16 non-structural and 4 structural proteins, among which some are necessary for entry into the host cell and replication. At the infection stage, the virus attaches itself to the cell with a spike glycoprotein (protein S), which is located in the outer envelope. This protein consists of two subunits, responsible for cell attachment and subsequent fusion (membrane protein, angiotensin-converting enzyme 2. The ability to bind the virus to the ACE2 membrane receptor. The target of the binding is the cellular which is much stronger for SARS-CoV-2 compared to SARS-CoV, which has the same binding site (Liu *et al.,* 2020). Protein S is hydrolyzed by endosomal proteases which results in membrane fusion.) Both the receptor itself and the proteases cutting spike protein are potential therapeutic targets. After fusion with a human cell, the virus releases its nucleotide into the cytoplasm and a number of molecular mechanisms are involved to produce the new RNA of the virus and the proteins that form its envelope. Key proteins involved in the replication and proliferation of the virus are an attractive target for antiviral compounds. Proteases, including papain-like protease and chymotrypsin-like protease are identified as the most important targets. In view of the high similarity of SARS-CoV-2 with SARS-CoV and MERS-CoV, the mechanism of action of compounds of plant origin may be similar.

Table 2: Bioactive compounds and their antiviral activity

Plant	*Active compounds*	*Virus type*	*Mechanism*
Green tea	Epigallocatechin gallate, epicatechingallate and gallocatechin-3-gallate	SARS-CoV-2	Interaction with catalytic residues of major protease
Brown algae *Sergas-sumspinuligerum*	1,3,5-Trihydroxybenzene	Inhibits major protease (M^{pro})	Brown algae *Sergassumspinuligerum*
Broussonetiapa-pyrifera	Polyphenols	SARS-CoV	Inhibition of cysteine proteases CoV
Brown algae *Ecklonia cava*	Phlorotannins i.e. dieckol	Inhibits SARS-CoV $3CL^{pro}$	Brown algae *Ecklonia cava*
Green tea	Epigallocatechin gallate (EGCg)	Bovine coronavirus (BCV)	EGCg works in the first stage of viral infection, the interaction between EGCg and BCV spiked glycoprotein
Sambucus nigra	Flavonoid anthocyanins lectins	Avian infectious bronchitis virus (IBV)	Inhibition of virus replication
Sambucus FormosanaNakai	Phenolic acids: caffeic acid, chlorogenic acid and gallic acid	HCoV-NL63	Inhibition of the replication of HCoV-NL63 in a cell-type independent manner
Sambucus FormosanaNakai	Flavonoids: herbacetin, isobavachalcone, quercetin 3-β-d-glucoside and helichrysetin	MERS- CoV	Inhibits MERS-CoV 3C-like protease ($3CL^{pro}$)

The potential use of plant extracts containing polyphenols to inhibit Covid-19-inducing corona virus: Literatures

The lack of Covid-19-oriented conventional therapeutic agents (vaccines, antibiotics) enforces the use of broad-spectrum antibiotics as well as widely known antiviral and corticosteroids. Supportive therapies, based on the agents of natural origin are also a solution of sorts. Extracts from natural products are a rich source of active compounds that can be used against corona virus.

Herbal extracts from traditional Chinese medicine plants *Cibotium barometz, Gentiana scabra, Dioscorea batatas, Cassia tora and Taxillus chinensis* were found to inhibit SARS-CoV replication (Wen *et al.,* 2011). The development of agents that inhibit coronavirus-associated respiratory syndrome (SARS-CoV) is important for both prevention and re-emergence of the disease. Wen *et al.,* (2011) investigated over 200 extracts from Chinese medicinal herbs for inhibition of SARS coronavirus. Cellular tests were conducted that investigate SARS-CoV induced cytopathogenic effect (CPE) on Vero E6 cells under in vitro conditions. Herbal extracts, from *Gentianae radix, Dioscoreaerhizoma, Cassiae Semen* and *Loranthi Ramus* (designated as GSH, DBM, CTH and TCH, respectively) and *Rhizoma Cibotii* (designated as CBE and CBM) in the concentrations from 25 to 200 ìg/ml proved to have potential inhibition effect on SARS-CoV. The concentrations of six extracts inhibited Vero E6 cell proliferation V (CC50) and virus replication (EC50) by 50%. The obtained selective index values (SI = CC50/EC50) for the most effective extracts from *RhizomaCibotii*, *Gentianae radix*, *Dioscoreaerhizoma*, *Cassiae Semen* and *Loranthi Ramus* and extracts were >59.4,> 57.5,> 62.1,> 59.4 and >92.9, respectively.

RhizomaCibotii and *Gentiana scabra* showed the most significant inhibition of SARS-CoV 3CL^{pro} activity. The IC50 values were 39 ìg/ml and 44 ìg/ml, respectively. Herbal extracts have been shown to have the potential as candidates for the development of SARS drugs or preventive preparations. Bioflavonoid from *Torreya nucifera* inhibited the replication of SARS-CoV3CL a research on the inhibitors among botanical sources of SARS-CoV 3CL. The authors studied ethanol extract from leaves of *Torreya nucifera*, a medicinal plant traditionally used in Asia. SARS-CoV 3CL inhibitory activity (62% at 100 ìg/ml) was found to be high. The authors identified eight diterpenoids and four bioflavonoid by fluorescence resonance energy transfer analysis as potential inhibitors of the virus. Biflavone amentoflavone (IC50 = 8.3 μM) was the most effective against the virus. Also the activity of flavones (apigenin, luteolin and quercetin) was investigated. IC50 values were 280.8, 20.2 and 23.8 μM, respectively. The binding energy values by the molecular docking study confirmed the results of enzymatic tests. The stronger activity was related to the presence of the apigenin moiety at the C-30 position of flavones, since biflavone had an effect on 3CL inhibitory.

The antiviral activity of ethyl acetate extract from *Houttuynia cordata* Thunb. containing quercetin, quercitrin and cyanserine in mouse corona virus and dengue virus infections (Chiow *et al.,* 2016) in *in vitro* tests. The flavonoids found in the extract (quercetin, quercitrin and rutin) were tested in terms of their efficiency against mouse coronavirus and dengue virus in virus neutralisation tests and acute oral toxicity in C57BL/6 mice. The plant extract inhibited viral infectivity for up to 6 days. Since the antiviral activity of some flavonoids is well known, the authors used a flavonoids library to study inhibitory compounds against the MERS-CoV 3C-like protease. The following compounds were found to block the enzymatic activity of MERS-CoV 3CL: herbacetin, isobavachalcone, quercetin 3-â-d-glucoside and helichristetine. The researchers conducted model tests on the binding of four flavonoids by the fluorescence-based tryptophan method. As a result, flavonol and chalcone were found to bind to the MERS-CoV $3CL^{pro}$ catalytic site. It was noticed that flavonoids derivatives with hydrophobic or carbohydrate groups attached to their core structures inhibit the virus. Such flavonoids can be used as templates to develop potential MERS-CoV 3CL inhibitors.

Here is provided a broad spectrum of information on the use of phytochemicals found in medicinal plants for the inhibition of corona virus family. Plant based foods are rich in Prebiotic which helps to improve our gut health and boost up immunity. Neutraceutical acts as super food and provides better health with the combination of food and natural medicine. This review also provides a glimpse of little herbal food and its role in health. Green tea, flavonoids and polyphenols are very effective phytochemical which inhibits the growth of virus. Indian herbs and traditional foods are very rich in its medicinal importance. MERS, SARS, and COVID-19 are infectious disease and spread due to the virus. Plant based phytochemicals are helpful against virus thus protect us from infection. Many types of herbal medicines are beneficial for boosting immunity and fighting against the virus.

We all must be aware of it that consuming prebiotic, probiotics, neutraceutical, and phytochemical in our daily diet will help in fighting with virus and boosting up immunity. Despite many unknowns, scientific research unambiguously indicates that plant extracts inhibit the life cycle of corona virus. Plant extracted phytochemical have high potential in the development of functional foods enriched with polyphenols of plant origin or even pharmaceutical preparations. It seems that the introduction of plant preparations into food and clinical practice should be relatively fast, because those are preparations of natural origin, obtained from plants authorised as herbs and food. It is worth mentioning that the benefit of using these preparations is highly safe for patients and have no known side effects.

References

1. Arlene Semeco, *et. al.* on June 08, 2016- Health line.
2. Breuer *et. al.* and Rademaker A.W.(1997). Short chain fatty acid rectal irritation for left sided ulcerative colitis: a randomized, placebo controlled trail. Gut, 40(4). 485-491.
3. Chen, L., Li, J., Luo, C., Liu, H., Xu, W., Chen, G., ... Jiang, H. (2006). Binding interaction of quercetin-3-β-galactoside and its synthetic derivatives with SARS-CoV 3CLpro: Structure-activity relationship studies reveal salient pharmacophore features. Bioorganic and Medicinal Chemistry, 14(24), 8295–8306.https://doi.org/10.1016/j.bmc.2006.09.014.
4. Chen, C. J., Michaelis, M., Hsu, H. K., Tsai, C. C., Yang, K. D., Wu, Y. C., ... Doerr, H. W. (2008). Toona sinensis Roem tender leaf extract inhibits SARS coronavirus replication. Journal of Ethnophar.
5. J Food Sci Technol. 2012 Apr; 49(2): 173–183. Published online 2011 Feb 26. Doi: 10.1007/s13197-011-0269-4
6. K. Chojnacka A. *et. al.* (2020). Phytochemicals containing biologically active polyphenols as an effective agent against Covid-19-inducing coronavirus. J. Fuctional Food. 1-8.
7. Mahmood, M. S., Mártinez, J. L., Aslam, A., Rafique, A., Vinet, R., Laurido, C., Ali, S. (2016). Antiviral effects of green tea (Camellia sinensis) against pathogenic viruses inhuman and animals (a mini-review). In African Journal of Traditional, Complementary and Alternative Medicines (Vol. 13, Issue 2, pp. 176–184).
8. M. Mukai, T. Furukawa, S. & Ohori, H. (2005). Inhibitory effects of epi-gallocatechin gallate on the propagation of bovine coronavirus in Madin-Darby bovine kidney cells. Animal Science Journal, 76(5), 507–512.
9. Meyers, K. J., Swiecki, T. J., & Mitchell, A. E. (2007). An exploratory study of the nutritional composition of tanoak (Lithocarpusdensiflorus) acorns after potassiumphosphonatetreatment.https.
10. Nguyen,T. T. H., Woo, H. J., Kang, H. K., Nguyen, V. D., Kim, Y. M., Kim, D. W., Kim, D. (2012). Flavonoid-mediated inhibition of SARS coronavirus 3C-like protease expressed in Pichia pastoris.Biotechnology Letters, 34(5), 831–8.
11. Remely *et.al.* A ,nd Haslberger, 4G; (2014). Effect of short chain fatty acid producing bacteria on epigenetic regulation of FFA R3 in type 2 diabetes and obesity. Gene: 573(1). 85-92.

Index

D

E

F

T

U

V

W

Z